The Everything Thyroid Disease Book

By: James M. Lowrance © 2011

I0449116

INTRODUCTION:

This comprehensive thyroid information resource contains 61 chapters, divided into three easy-to-navigate sections.

SECTION ONE: "Hypothyroidism" – an under active thyroid gland, accounts for 80% of thyroid disorder cases and this section contains 17 chapters dedicated to the most common thyroid disorder that exists. All aspects regarding hypothyroid conditions are addressed in easy-to-understand language. Anyone from a novice reader to a medical professional can benefit from the compiled information.

SECTION TWO: "Hyperthyroidism" – an overactive thyroid gland, accounts for 20% of thyroid disease cases. Within the 10-chapters, the most common cause - Graves' disease is also addressed, as well as complications, including Thyroid Eye Disease, toxic diffuse goiter, hot nodules, myopathy of the muscles and a hyperthyroid condition that can be life-threatening (i.e. thyroid storm).

SECTION THREE: "Thyroid Disease" – in general, containing 34 chapters covering everything about disorders, conditions and imbalances of the thyroid gland. Medical professionals and laypersons can benefit from the extensively- researched and well-confirmed information. Included, is information on thyroid antibodies (autoimmunity), goiters, thyroid nodules, cancer, risk factors for developing thyroid disease, types of thyroiditis, coping with a diseased thyroid gland, famous people with thyroid disease (like Oprah Winfrey) and much, much more.

TABLE OF CONTENTS:

SECTION ONE: **Everything about Hypothyroidism**

CHAPTER THIRTYFOUR
Online Thyroid Support and Information
Coping For Patients on the World Wide Web

SECTION ONE: **Everything about Hypothyroidism**

CHAPTER ONE

Hypothyroidism Basic Facts

Under active Thyroid Gland General Information

The American Association of Clinical Endocrinologists (AACE) estimates that approximately 27-million Americans suffer thyroid diseases and up to 13-million cases remain undiagnosed. Hypothyroid conditions account for about 80% of abnormal thyroid function cases. There are varied symptoms, causes, diagnostic methods and treatments for hypothyroidism.

When a person experiences hypothyroidism, meaning his or her thyroid hormone production has decreased to abnormally low levels (low T3 and/or T4) this results in the metabolism becoming slowed down. The resulting effects are signs and symptoms affecting every area of the body with the severity of them depending on how advanced the hypothyroidism is.

Major Causes of Hypothyroidism

Hypothyroidism can have causes that are "primary" (in the gland) or "secondary" (indirectly affecting the gland). The number one cause of hypothyroidism, worldwide is iodine deficiency which is due to the fact that third world countries (less industrialized) account for most of the world population and are areas where iodine is lacking in their diets. The thyroid gland depends on iodine for production of thyroid hormones. Part of this lack comes from their not having iodized salt as we do, who live in the more advanced countries of the world where iodized salt is more easily attainable.

Industrialized countries have "thyroid autoimmunity" as the most common cause of hypothyroidism. This would also be referred to as "chronic autoimmune thyroiditis", with most cases falling under the "Hashimoto's thyroiditis" umbrella.

Thyroid removal surgeries or procedures, in which part of the thyroid gland is removed as treatment for hyperthyroidism (overactive) or to remove thyroid nodules or large goiters, can also result in the need following, to replace thyroid hormone levels that become low afterward.

Other less-common causes of hypothyroidism include pregnancies and problems involving the major glands in the brain that regulate hormone production in the thyroid gland. These are the "hypothalamus" (sends TRH to the pituitary gland) and the "pituitary" (sends TSH to the thyroid, in response to TRH). These glands work in a continuous loop unless disrupted by tumors that can develop within them with hypothyroidism being the end result when the process is hindered, also called "Central Hypothyroidism".

Hypothyroid Symptoms

A slowed metabolism from hypothyroidism can cause an array of symptoms. These include:

• joint and muscle aches

• depression

- fatigue and low energy

- dry skin

- hair loss

- constipation

- weight gain

- water retention

- swelling in the body (edema)

- slowed heart rate and breathing

- heavier menstrual cycles

- elevated cholesterol

- goiter and changes in appetite

Symptom severity varies depending on the progression of hypothyroidism.

Diagnosis

Most cases of hypothyroidism are diagnosed through medical blood lab testing. A doctor will order a thyroid panel that includes several tests or he will possibly order a single test. These tests will measure the T3 and/or T4 thyroid hormones levels and/or the TSH level (Thyroid Stimulating Hormone).

With hypothyroidism, the T3 and/or T4 levels will decrease to low levels, while the TSH will increase to a high level. This is due to TSH being the hormone as mentioned earlier, that stimulates hormone production in the thyroid gland and when the gland is not producing enough, the pituitary increases TSH to an abnormally high level. In some cases, TSH will be the test that detects hypothyroidism earlier than any other tests.

Less commonly used tests to detect hypothyroidism are the "Radioactive Iodine Scan" and the "Radioactive Iodine Uptake Test". The first mentioned scan is done by administering radioactive iodine to a patient and taking radiology camera images to see how evenly the thyroid gland is absorbing iodine. The second mentioned test does not involve imaging but is a measure of how much iodine is being absorbed by the thyroid gland.

If the thyroid gland fails to absorb an adequate amount of iodine, hypothyroidism may be diagnosed. These tests are more commonly used to determine causes of hyperthyroidism (overactive gland) when excessive amounts of iodine are absorbed and to detect thyroid nodules (tumors) when iodine is absorbed unevenly in the gland.

Treatment

The goal of treatment for hypothyroidism is to increase low levels of thyroid hormone via a dose of prescribed replacement hormone. Doctors often prescribe synthetic T4 hormone drugs but some do prescribe combinations of T4 and T3 that come in either synthetic or natural brands. There is ongoing controversy in regard to which type of replacement hormone works best but the importance of the hypothyroid therapy lies in how well it is monitored and optimized.

The goal is to accomplish best possible symptom relief for patients, with dose adjustments made to restore bodily metabolism to the best possible level. This is done by monitoring the dose via repeat blood tests at approximately 8-week intervals, to measure the TSH, T4 and T3 levels. Once the proper levels are reached, TSH may be the only repeat blood test that is needed, with retests repeated about 2 to 4 times yearly.

In chapters that follow, more detail will be given to the subject of thyroid hormone replacement therapy, the treatment for cases of hypothyroidism.

CHAPTER TWO

Primary and Secondary Hypothyroid Disorders

Direct and Indirect Causes of an Under active Thyroid Gland

Most cases of hypothyroidism are due to problems within the thyroid gland but there are other causes that indirectly cause under-functioning of the gland.

Thyroid disease is a primary cause of hypothyroidism, meaning it is a problem within the thyroid gland itself. Secondary causes of hypothyroidism would be those that do not originate within the gland but are other problems within the body that indirectly affect thyroid hormone levels.

Primary Causes

Thyroid autoimmunity - is an immune system response, in which auto-antibodies are created to attack thyroid proteins and is the most common cause of hypothyroidism in industrialized countries. In addition to causing destruction of thyroid tissue over time that result in the gland under-functioning, normal thyroid tissue is also taken over by abnormal tissue. Eventually, the gland can no longer absorb iodine from things in the diet, to produce thyroid hormone from. This may also include development of thyroid nodules (small tumors) that take up space within the gland, so that there is less normal tissue for normal thyroid functioning.

Other primary causes – include injuries to the thyroid gland that diminish its ability to function normally and glands that are not fully developed at birth or following birth. If for example, a person is in a severe car accident that causes trauma to the throat, the thyroid gland can be directly damaged and once this occurs, any resulting hypothyroidism would be a problem within the gland. People who are born with only partial thyroid glands or small inadequate ones that do not develop as they become adults, can experience hypothyroidism which would also be a problem originating within the gland itself.

Secondary Causes

Biochemical hypothyroidism – are cases in which a chemical element needed by the thyroid gland is lacking or the gland is damaged by a drug or other chemical that is harmful to the body or hinders thyroid function. Iodine deficiency is in this category and occurs when there is inadequate iodine consumed in the diet. The thyroid is highly dependent on this chemical element that is used by the gland to produce hormones that regulate metabolism and so iodine deficiency causes the thyroid to hypo-function. An example of chemical damage to the thyroid and resulting hypothyroidism would be when drinking water has been contaminated with radioactive chemicals and results in cell destruction within the gland.

Failure of major endocrine brain glands – is a condition often referred to as "Central Hypothyroidism", meaning the brain-center is failing to regulate the thyroid gland. The two master glands that stimulate the thyroid to operate at normal levels are the hypothalamus and pituitary glands. The hypothalamus sends TRH (thyrotrophin releasing hormone) to the pituitary gland, which in turn sends TSH (thyroid stimulating hormone), also called "thyrotrophin" to the thyroid gland, which completes the process by supplying the body with thyroid hormones. A failure on the part of either master gland, due to tumors within them or disease processes affecting them, results in secondary/central hypothyroidism.

Other secondary causes – include women who develop under-functioning thyroid glands as a result of pregnancy, also referred to as "postpartum hypothyroidism". Certain types of diseases can also affect thyroid function, including those affecting other glands in the endocrine system (hormone producing). Chronic stress and severe emotional disorders can cause the T3 thyroid hormone specifically to become low. This less-common condition is referred to as "Euthyroid Sick Syndrome" or "low T3 Syndrome" and is a secondary cause that usually only requires short term treatment to resolve it.

Patients who are diagnosed with hypothyroidism should request that their doctors inform them of the cause of their thyroid disorder. This may require additional diagnostic testing but will help better-educate patients about the disease that is affecting them.

CHAPTER THREE

Hashimoto's Disease and Hypothyroid Treatment

Hypothyroidism from Autoimmune Thyroiditis

Hashimoto's is an autoimmune type of thyroiditis that leads to hypothyroidism. While there is no cure for the disease, the resulting hypothyroidism can be treated.

Hashimoto's thyroiditis affects approximately 14-million Americans and is 7 times more common in women than in men. It is the leading cause of hypothyroidism in industrialized countries and the second leading cause of an under-active thyroid gland in people worldwide, taking second place to iodine deficiency hypothyroidism. While there is no cure for this autoimmune thyroid disease, there is treatment for the hypothyroidism it causes.

Hashimoto's is an Autoimmune Disease

With Hashimoto's thyroiditis, auto-antibodies including the "anti-thyroidperoxidase" and the "anti-thyroglobulin" are created by the immune system to attack the thyroid gland. For reasons yet to be fully understood by medical research, the immune system will at times target a natural part of the body and will relentlessly attack it. There are a number of theories including viral agents, allergens or intolerant foods entering the body as causes of autoimmune responses.

Viruses that cannot be fully eliminated by the immune system for example may result in it turning on the body to destroy tissues that contain the virus. For whatever reason the body turns on itself with autoimmune diseases, it causes a mistaken identity. These natural tissues, organs, glands, muscles or joints are recognized as enemies in the body and are attacked. When the immune system is operating properly, it will create antibodies only to attack unnatural invaders that can potentially cause illness or disease in the body. With Hashimoto's, the immune system has turned on the thyroid gland to destroy it as a mistaken enemy.

Hashimoto's leads to Hypothyroidism

As the killer cells called "thyroid antibodies" begin to destroy natural thyroid gland protein-cells, it begins to cause death to the gland at a gradual rate. Antibody levels can vary among Hashimoto's patients and those with very high elevations of thyroid antibodies may see faster cell destruction and damage to the gland. As the damage occurs, the gland becomes less capable of producing thyroid hormone to regulate the metabolism of the body.

The resulting condition of slowed-metabolism is called "hypothyroidism". Many patients with the disease experience few or no symptoms until hypothyroidism begins to set in. Mild cases of an under-active thyroid from Hashimoto's can begin to cause symptoms of fatigue, weight gain, fluid retention (myxedema), dry skin and brittle hair, depression and/or anxiety and constipation.

Treatment for Hashimoto's

This autoimmune thyroiditis is irreversible in the vast majority of cases and medical research has not found a cure for autoimmune diseases in-general nor do they understand why they go into remission in rare cases. The treatment that will need to be administered is for the resulting hypothyroidism caused by the disease. Once symptoms and/or lab tests reveal that the thyroid gland has become under-active, thyroid hormone replacement therapy is the treatment that is administered.

Some medical sources also believe that hormone replacement may help to reduce thyroid antibody levels over time. Other medical research articles state that supplementing Hashimoto's patients with "selenium" may also help to reduce high elevations of thyroid antibodies but the dose should be at a proper level and monitored by a treating physician.

CHAPTER FOUR

Risks for Developing Hypothyroidism

Factors Contributing to an Under active Thyroid Gland

There are genetic factors and other natural events that occur in life that place people at higher risk for the development of thyroid disease.

Thyroid diseases can affect anyone at any point in their lives there are however things that can add to the already present potential or probability that a person will develop a disease or disorder affecting thyroid hormone balance. With 80% of thyroid problems being in the hypothyroidism (under-functioning) category, this is the area that will be addressed in the following subheadings.

Being Female

If a person is female, rather than male, her chance for developing hypothyroidism has already increased at least five-fold. While statistics vary, it can be reasonably stated that thyroid disease in-general is no less than five times more common in women than in men. The female endocrine system (hormone producing) is more complicated than that of males due to there being the reproductive organs present, for giving birth and that experience the cycling each month from the age of puberty that signals times of high fertility (menses).

The fertility cycles that occur in females cause wide swings in the levels of sex, adrenal and thyroid hormones and may be the reason hormone imbalances and diseases develop more often affecting the endocrine systems of women. The endocrine system as a whole works in unison or what might be referred to as "a loop" or "in sync" and so changes in the levels of one endocrine hormone, can affect the levels of others.

It may be possible that these changes in endocrine hormones trigger an immune system response in some women (autoimmune disease), in which antibodies are created to attack the glands causing these wide fluctuations. When, the thyroid gland is affected it is referred to as "thyroid autoimmunity". As women enter the age when reproduction responsiveness slows down (menopause), this too may contribute to thyroid hormone imbalance. Some medical sources are of the opinion that birth control pills may contribute to development of thyroid problems as well.

Being the Offspring of Parents with Thyroid Disease

If one or both of a person's parents have thyroid disease, this places him or her at high risk for developing thyroid problems of their own. According to Hossein Gharib, M.D., a member of the AACE (American Association of Clinical Endocrinologists) and a medical research professor at the Mayo Medical College, 50% of thyroid disorder parents will have offspring that inherit the gene responsible for thyroid disease development. Some medical sources state that thyroid problems can be present in children of thyroid disease parents, at birth or in early childhood but will not be detectable in most of them until about the age of 35 or 40 years.

Pregnancy

Approximately two percent of women, who become pregnant, develop under-active thyroid glands. Thyroid disorders during pregnancy can range from temporary thyroiditis to permanent hypothyroidism requiring lifelong treatment (25% are permanent). Thyroid disorders can manifest during pregnancy or following (postpartum) and estimates state that up to 10% of cases develop within a year after giving birth. Most cases involve under-active thyroid glands with only about 1% being cases of hyperthyroidism (overactive).

Senior Citizens

Generally, thyroid disease occurs most commonly in the general population at between the ages of 35 and 40. Those who do not develop thyroid problems due to other factors as detailed in the previous subheadings can still develop age-related hypothyroidism as they reach their senior years.

Approximately 15% of women develop hypothyroidism by the age of 60 years and approximately 8% of men do so by the same age.

These cases are generally not due to a disease process but are a result of a diminished ability for thyroid glands in the elderly to produce the needed levels of hormones. Their glands are in-essence experiencing a degree of atrophy, meaning shrinkage and a diminished ability to function at pre-senior age levels. If thyroid symptoms do not appear in males or females by age 40, it is still recommended that blood testing of thyroid hormones be conducted to rule out developing thyroid disease.

CHAPTER FIVE

Varied Effectiveness of Thyroid Hormone Therapy

Optimized Treatment for Hypothyroidism

Hypothyroid patients deserve specialized treatment from treating doctors who monitor and adjust their thyroid hormone dose to best possible symptom-relieving levels.

For patients with hypothyroidism, thyroid hormone replacement therapy effectiveness is very important. The more symptom relief that can be experienced, the better patients are able to carry on normal activities of work, school and leisure activities. In other words, they will regain the best quality-of-life possible. This is where the importance in securing the best possible doctor for administering the treatment comes in, as well as his or her ability to best optimize that therapy.

The fact is, that thyroid hormone therapies vary in effectiveness, depending upon the type that is being administered and how well it is being monitored by the treating doctor via repeat blood lab testing. Most hypothyroid patients need dose adjustments to bring their thyroid hormones back to the proper level and eventually finely-tuned further to an optimal level.

Each patient has that target level that brings them the most symptom relief or what might be called their "set-point". This level of treatment varies among patients and further demonstrates the importance in a quality thyroid doctor, meaning one who specializes in optimizing treatment for hypothyroid patients.

Finding the Right Type of Thyroid Hormone Dose

Most patients are started on a dose of thyroxine to treat their hypothyroidism, which is a T4 only hormone dose, usually prescribed in the synthetic form. The two major thyroid hormones that regulate the body's metabolism are the T4 and T3 and we depend on the body's natural process of converting the needed T3 from the T4. For some patients this does not happen adequately and this problem is referred to as "impaired conversion".

The treating doctor also needs to be aware of these possibilities and to know how to monitor for them. If a patient does experience impaired conversion, the doctor needs to be willing to add T3 hormone to the patient's replacement therapy dose. Some doctors start patients on T4/T3 combination hormone doses because they believe it is more effective in some patients than a T4-only dose.

The Importance of Repeat Blood Test Monitoring

To fully monitor the hormone therapy of newly treated hypothyroid patients, a doctor needs to order full thyroid panels that include TSH, T4 and T3, the "free levels" of the later two being the better versions (as opposed to the "total levels") according to many thyroid specialists and endocrinologists. This more thorough monitoring for at least the first few blood retests will better evaluate the thyroid hormone therapy and help the doctor to know what changes are needed in the dose or type of thyroid hormone that is needed.

If this type of specialized treatment is not offered to hypothyroid patients, many may potentially remain in a state of unrelieved hypothyroid symptoms and the opportunity will be missed to restore a better quality-of-life to them.

CHAPTER SIX

T4 and T3 Hypothyroid Treatment Options

Hormone Treatments for an Under active Thyroid

Some hypothyroid patients are successfully treated with a T4 thyroid hormone replacement dose. Others may also need T3 hormone added to their treatment.

The majority of diagnosed hypothyroid patients are prescribed T4 replacement hormone medications. These are types/brands that replace low thyroxine levels, which is the T4 hormone that also converts into the other major thyroid hormone called T3 (triiodothyronine). Brands of thyroxine are also referred to as "levothyroxine sodium" and include the following brands.

- Synthroid

- Levoxyl

- Levothroid

- Unithroid

Thyroxine-T4 Replacement Therapy and Impaired Conversion

Once a dose of T4-only replacement hormone is taken, the treated patient and treating doctor must depend on the T4 to successfully convert into T3 as it is needed in the body. In the majority of hypothyroid patients, this occurs adequately as needed; however, in a small percent of patients, they will experience "impaired conversion". The lack of T3 being converted will keep them in a state of hypothyroidism or what might be referred to as "Low T3 Syndrome". Monitoring for impaired conversion requires the treating doctor to retest the patient's blood levels of both T4 and T3 to see if proper conversion is occurring. This phenomenon will be mentioned further in chapters that follow.

Combination T4 and T3 Replacement Therapy

Some doctors, who treat hypothyroidism, prefer to prescribe combination T4 and T3 thyroid hormone replacement medications. They believe this type of therapy is superior to T4-only replacement whether impaired conversion is an issue or not. Brands of combination T4 and T3 thyroid hormone drugs include the following.

- Thyrolar

- Armour Thyroid

• Nature-Throid

• Westhroid

Most cases of hypothyroidism are caused by types of "thyroid autoimmunity", also referred to as chronic thyroiditis (i.e. Hashimoto's, Riedel's and Ord's). Auto-antibodies sent from the immune system, to attack thyroid proteins that convert iodine into thyroid hormones. Because of this, there can be a significant percent of hormone being blocked from conversion and this will cause the T3 level to remain at sub-optimal level, even when the dose of T4 coming into the body is adequate. While the T3 may remain within normal range, it will stay slightly below the mid-level of normal values or at lower normal.

The Treatment Goal for T4 and T3

Some hypothyroid patients may experience better symptom relief if both the T4 and T3 are at mid-range or higher-normal. This can be accomplished in most patients who are placed on a T4-only dose but for those whose ratio of T4 to T3 is not remaining balanced at mid-range or above, a combination of T4 and T3 thyroid hormone dose may offer the solution. This too is better determined by testing both thyroid hormone levels in treated hypothyroid patients. Testing the TSH alone (Thyroid Stimulating Hormone) may not detect a low T3 level in some cases either. This pituitary gland hormone may test at normal range even if the T4-only is at proper level but the T3 is not.

Triiodothyronine-T3 Replacement Therapy

A dose of T3-only (Liothyronine Sodium) is usually restricted to cases of "Low T3 Syndrome" or what is also commonly referred to as "Euthyroid Sick Syndrome" or

"Wilson's Syndrome". This condition of low T3 can occur in heart disease patients, in athletes who undergo strenuous training and in people with severe depression or chronic stress. It can also occur in cancer patients and in other cases of chronic or inflammatory diseases.

A T3 dose of thyroid hormone replacement may be administered to patients with this type of hypothyroidism caused by low T3 levels. The cause of the hypothyroidism will also be treated or corrected and if significant improvement occurs, the T3 replacement therapy may only be needed temporarily (short-term).

Doses of T3-only hormone medications are also sometimes added to T4 doses in hypothyroid patients so that the treating doctor can choose the specific ratio of T4 to T3 he deems necessary for the patient. The most recognized brand of T3 hormone available is called "Cytomel", manufactured by King Pharmaceuticals. Some doctors may also refer their hypothyroid patients to compounding pharmacies who combine the needed ratio of T4 to T3 into a specially manufactured dose, tailored to the individual patient's needs.

CHAPTER SEVEN

Hypothyroid Therapy Adjustment Symptoms

Thyroid Hormone Replacement Side Effects

Some patients who start hormone replacement therapy for hypothyroidism will experience adjustment symptoms to the new dose.

Most newly treated hypothyroid patients see these adjustment symptoms resolve after a few weeks on their thyroid medication. Many patients require one or more dose increases following an initial starting dose to elevate their thyroid hormone levels to a proper level. This process can take several months before an adequate or optimal treatment level is achieved.

How Doctors Monitor Treatment

A new dose is monitored via follow up blood retests as previously mentioned and if it is found to be lower than is needed to adequately treat a patient's hypothyroidism, it is increased. In some cases a dose increase may be needed several times to reach the desired level and in some cases a dose decrease may be needed (a lower dose) if levels test abnormally high at some point.

If it is several months between a scheduled blood retest and a patient is experiencing symptoms that indicate the need for a dose adjustment, the treating doctor may retest the levels earlier than scheduled and adjust the patient's dose accordingly.

If a patient's dose is too low, they may experience one or more of the following hypothyroid symptoms:

• constipation

• depression

• fatigue

• excessive need for sleep

• dry skin

• joint and muscle aches

If a patient's dose is too high, they may experience hyperthyroid symptoms that include the following:

• rapid heart rate

• diarrhea

• anxiety and nervousness

• sweating

• tremors

• insomnia

• muscle weakness

Types of Thyroid Hormone Doses

Adjustment symptoms may occur more often in patients who take replacement hormone brands that contain the T3 thyroid hormone (it is at least five times more potent that T4); however, patients who take a T4-only hormone may also experience dose-adjustment type symptoms. It takes approximately eight weeks to see a new dose level-out in the body and to start doing it's job properly.

The following are types of prescribed thyroid hormone medications that are administered to hypothyroid patients and that require adjustment to them in the body.

• synthetic T4

• synthetic T3

• combination synthetic T4 and T3

• combination natural (animal derived) T4 and T3

• compounded (varied ratio) mix of T4 and T3

How the Thyroid Gland Responds to Replacement Therapy

Many patients, who do experience adjustment type symptoms to thyroid hormone replacement, will either see worsening hypothyroid symptoms or may have some mild to moderate hyperthyroid type symptoms. Either type usually resolves after a few weeks. This happens because the thyroid gland responds to hormone coming into the body from the outside, by shutting off part or all of its own production of hormone. When this happens, the body sometimes reaches a break-even point before improvement of hypothyroid symptoms begins.

Other patient's thyroid glands are slower to cut back production of hormone, as the dose comes into the body, so will experience hyperthyroid type symptoms for a brief period of time. These two scenarios can also depend on how much damage has occurred in the thyroid gland from antibody-destruction, meaning the attack from auto-antibodies being sent to the gland from the immune system (thyroid autoimmunity).

If a patient's thyroid gland has been damaged from highly elevated antibody levels, as a dose of thyroid hormone is administered, their own gland will begin shutting down (atrophy) and adjustment symptoms may occur in the body.

This might also be referred to as "side effects" from the starting dose.

Suppressing the TSH Level

According to the U.S. NIH (National Institutes of Health) a hormone replacement dose for hypothyroidism needs to suppress the blood TSH level (pituitary hormone that reflects thyroid levels) down to between 0.5 and 3.0 mIU/L over time (average TSH normal range: 0.5 to 5.0 mIU/L) and the T4 and T3 need to be raised to around mid-range or upper-normal (ranges vary among testing labs).

This can take time and possibly several dose adjustments monitored at eight-week intervals by blood retests of TSH, T4 & T3. Most doctors prefer to start patients on a low dose and increase it upward (titrate) until it reaches the proper level to sufficiently treat a patient's hypothyroidism.

CHAPTER EIGHT

Distinguishing between Diagnostic and Treatment TSH

A Narrower Normal Values Range for Treating Hypothyroidism

The normal reference range for Thyroid Stimulating Hormone (diagnostic TSH) is not the same as the range used by most doctors for treating under active thyroid glands.

The goal of thyroid hormone therapy to treat patients with hypothyroid conditions is to suppress their elevated TSH levels, down to a lower normal level. As the TSH is suppressed, the thyroid hormone levels (T4 and T3) will rise in response to corrected levels (from low to normal). Keeping TSH at a higher normal level, even if that level remains within normal values, may not result in adequate treatment for some patients.

Diagnostic TSH Range

The normal values TSH range for detecting thyroid hormone imbalance at medical blood labs has a high-normal boundary and a low-normal boundary. Readings falling outside of those, even slightly, can indicate an existing thyroid hormone imbalance or one that is developing. The range will be fairly wide, so that less-than borderline cases do not appear to be abnormal readings, which can be misleading to a doctor, resulting in additional testing or follow-up monitoring that may not be necessary.

A blood lab for example may have a normal range for TSH, to diagnose thyroid dysfunction that is from 0.4 to 4.0, with readings that fall below 0.4 indicating thyroid hormone levels are elevating in the body and with readings rising above 4.0 indicating thyroid hormones are decreasing in the body. If readings are at either of the cut-off levels but not outside of them (borderline), these cases still merit follow up retesting because they may point to developing thyroid hormone imbalance. This is a fact stated by the U.S. National Institutes of Health.

Treatment TSH Range

When hypothyroidism is being treated, which can develop directly from a disease process or following treatment for hyperthyroidism, the goal is not simply to correct the TSH level back into the normal values range. The goal is rather to treat the hypothyroidism, so that TSH is at a level that also places the thyroid hormones at the proper level to relieve symptoms of hypothyroidism and to correct the patient's slow functioning metabolism.

A borderline high or higher-normal TSH level may not accomplish this; in fact some patients may require TSH to be suppressed to low-normal levels to properly increase the T4 and T3. Blood testing all three levels together can better help to determine where the TSH level needs to be.

TSH Range - Too wide at Some Labs

Both the AACE (American Association of Clinical Endocrinologists) and the NACB (National Academy of Clinical Biochemistry) have recommended that labs with wide TSH ranges, narrow those ranges to a level that detects more cases of developing thyroid hormone disorders. The AACE has expressed belief that TSH levels above "3.0" may indicate developing hypothyroidism, while the NACB states that the upper limit (high normal) TSH reference range may at some point need to be reduced to "2.5". This is based on their observance of the fact that 95% of euthyroid (normal thyroid function) individuals test between "0.4 and 2.5".

CHAPTER NINE

Thyroid Hormone Treatment Controversies

Issues of Debate Regarding Hypothyroid Therapies

The debate is ongoing as to which type hormone

replacement therapy is best. The answer is not actually a "one size fits all" one but one of patient-individuality.

Doctors who treat hypothyroidism should see each patient as an individual who needs monitored for both the effectiveness of the treatment and possible problems that might arise from the thyroid hormone replacement therapy. If a patient fails to experience satisfactory symptom relief, a trial of a different type of prescribed hormone might hold the answer to better treatment success.

Brand Favoritism In-Balance

Doctors should certainly form their opinions as to which thyroid hormone type or brand works better in the general population of hypothyroid patients. When a doctor however, highly favors a particular brand over all others, to the point of unwillingness to switch patients struggling with unresolved symptoms to trials of other types, this could result in missed opportunities for improved symptom-relief for individual patients who sometimes have unique treatment-needs.

Doctors should also be willing to consider suggestions by their patients, as to which thyroid hormone therapy they feel might be better suited for them. All available types require being prescribed by a treating doctor who will also monitor the treatment and a preference expressed by a patient for a particular type or brand does not change this fact. Doctors, who do not specialize in thyroid treatment or who are having problems treating patients with difficult cases, should also be willing to refer them to Thyroid Specialists or Endocrinologists when needed.

Does Synthetic T4 Restore Metabolism?

There has been very strong debate by advocates on both sides of the thyroid hormone brand issue, one being represented by proponents who feel natural brands of T4 and T3 combination are the best treatment-option for hypothyroidism, the other being proponents who believe synthetic T4-only to be the best treatment-option. Points that are often included in the debate include the view that both T4 and T3 are needed to restore normal metabolism in many hypothyroid patients.

In defense of thyroxine-only replacement therapy (not containing T3), it is often pointed out that once a proper dose-level of synthetic T4 is administered, the proof of how well the hormone is being used by the body can be seen in follow-up blood tests. These tests and retests can include one that also measures the Free T3 level which can determine if the patient's body is properly recognizing the hormone and converting it into the proper level of this more metabolically active hormone.

The other consideration is "symptom improvement" (including correction of elevated cholesterol levels) and if both of these factors are satisfactorily taking place, why would a patient or doctor want to see the type or brand of treatment switched? Trying to fix things that are not broken can sometimes cause more problems than solutions.

"T3 Does Not Add Benefit for Some Patients."

This type statement fits into the "one size fits all" category of debate-view and while it may be true in some cases it will not be true in all cases. One aspect that is often added to this argument against the addition of T3 hormone into a treatment for a hypothyroid patient is the fact that the hormone is fast-acting and has a shorter half-life than T4 has. The opinion therefore is that it is unstable in patients and causes spikes and crashes in T3 levels. The fact is however that treatment containing T3 is taken on a daily basis and this alone helps to keep levels stable.

Additionally, the same mentions in the previous subheading in regard to blood retests that monitor thyroid hormone replacement therapy also apply to therapies that include T3. If blood levels remain stable and symptom-relief is experienced, this should signal treatment success to both the patient and doctor.

There are also medical studies that have concluded that hypothyroid therapy in depressed patients with difficult to resolve depression symptoms, can benefit from the addition of T3 to their thyroid hormone replacement therapy. This too is a factor demonstrating patient-individuality and another consideration both patient and doctor should look at if this scenario involving depression exists in a patient.

Allergies and Intolerances

A small percent of patients placed on certain types of thyroid hormone whether synthetic or natural brands will have allergic or intolerant reactions to them. Many medications contain fillers that help manufactures process them into pill form or that help the drug to better absorb in the systems of patients who take them. These patients, whose systems recognize these fillers as allergens, will experience symptoms such as hives and stomach upset. This will require the treating doctor to switch the patient to a brand that is better tolerated.

Some thyroid hormone brands are derived from the glands of pigs (porcine source) and there are people who are intolerant to any type of pork or related products. In cases like these it may be either the synthetic or the natural brand that works better for these patients with sensitivities. Some natural brands of thyroid hormone are "hypoallergenic", meaning all know allergy-causing ingredients have been removed.

Generic Vs Major Brands

Some patients will see their doctors change their prescriptions from a major thyroid hormone brand, to a generic for insurance purposes or to save self-pay patients on their costs. Generics in all types of medications have been found to sometimes be slightly less potent when compared to major brands. In the case of thyroid hormone therapy, this can mean that the patient's T4 and T3 levels may drop slightly as a result of switching to a generic brand. This will require the treating doctor to increase the dose level to compensate for the different in potency.

With any switch of a thyroid hormone prescription, whether from synthetic to natural or from major brand to generic, patients need blood retested about eight weeks following the switch-over. If blood retesting is set at a longer interval of three to six months, the patient may experience a period of hypothyroid symptoms.

Additional Reasons for Brand Preferences

In addition to the aforementioned, there are other reasons some patients require a particular brand of thyroid hormone or who must be restricted from certain brands. Some patients for example, experience a less-common condition called "low T3 syndrome" that requires replacing only the T3 thyroid hormone until the condition resolves. The reverse can also be true, demonstrated by the fact that some hypothyroid patients are highly sensitive to T3 supplementation. They will have hyperthyroid type side effects from even low doses of oral dosing which in some cases may be due to another type of deficiency or hormone imbalance present in their bodies.

In other cases, a person's religious beliefs or convictions restrict the use of products made from certain animals. This can also be true of people who practice firm beliefs in the area of animal advocacy or who, are vegetarians. All of the preceding described reasons demonstrate the reasons for the existence of synthetic, natural and variation of T4 and T3 brands.

CHAPTER TEN

Optimizing Hypothyroidism Treatment Levels

TSH Monitoring of Thyroid Hormone Therapy

Most treated hypothyroid patients experience significant symptom relief and regain normal metabolism, while others experience difficulties with inadequate treatment.

Thyroid hormone replacement is simple to administer and requires that a patient take a daily dose of synthetic or natural thyroid hormone to restore bodily metabolism. While the method of treatment is simple, it is also important that a treating doctor is sensitive to the needs of individual patients. This demonstrates the importance in hypothyroid patients being treated by qualified thyroid doctors and in patients being fully communicative about progress and symptom-relief (or a lack in these) with their treating doctors.

Optimized Treatment Goals

It is a fact that there are doctors who specialize in thyroid treatments and those who do not. Those who do often have targeted treatment goals for patients, rather than simply treating them to get their thyroid hormone levels replaced back into the normal values range. The two major thyroid hormones that are monitored with hypothyroid therapy are the T4 and T3 levels. A low-normal thyroid hormone level or even one that is at about mid-range will not be optimal for some patients who instead need the levels at between mid-range and high-normal to experience significant symptom relief.

TSH Suppression

Looking at it from the point-of-view of the TSH level (pituitary hormone that reflects thyroid hormone levels), the goal of a replacement thyroid hormone dose is to suppress the elevated TSH level (elevates with hypothyroidism) back down to normal range. Some patients however, need a significantly suppressed TSH to cause thyroid hormones (T4 and T3) to rise slightly above mid-range in the body.

If the TSH normal values range at a blood lab is for example from "0.5 to 5.0IU/L", a thyroid hormone dose that only suppresses TSH down to "3.5" may not result in adequate increases in thyroid hormone levels or in the symptom relief that is needed by the patient. The U.S. National Institutes of Health states that hypothyroidism should be treated to place a patient's TSH level at between

"0.5 and 3.0 mIU/L". Levels such as "1.0" and "2.0" are within that treatment goal range.

Patient Individuality

The scenario addressed in the previous subheading is sometimes reversed and a hypothyroid patient may not need a significantly suppressed TSH for thyroid hormone levels to become optimized. Some patients in fact will experience mild, ongoing hyperthyroid (overactive) type symptoms if their TSH is suppressed below a "2.5" or "2.0". It is not always apparent as to why patients may vary in this area but could be due to differences in the functioning of their regulating brain glands (the master endocrine ones), or more specifically in how their pituitary function may vary slightly in response to thyroid hormone coming into the body from an outside source (the resulting TSH level).

Blood Retesting TSH and Thyroid Hormones

Detecting differences in the needs of individual patients may require blood testing their T4 and T3 levels in addition to TSH, to better evaluate how these levels all correlate. Once a doctor knows where the TSH level needs to fall within the treatment range to optimize a patient's thyroid hormone levels via a replacement dose, he can then blood retest using TSH-only. If TSH and thyroid hormones are not first evaluated together in follow up on hypothyroid therapy, opportunity to better optimize a patient's treatment might be missed.

CHAPTER ELEVEN

Thyroid Disease Related Depression

When Thyroid Treatment does not Relieve Depression

Thyroid treatments do not always successfully resolve the emotional symptoms of depression in all patients. Some need additional treatments or therapies administered.

Thyroid hormone imbalances are well-known for causing emotional and mood disorders including major depression. Both hypothyroid and hyperthyroid conditions have potential to cause symptoms of depression and/or anxiety. For some well-treated thyroid patients, their emotional symptoms persist and they need additional help with coping and symptom relief, through added medications or therapies.

Symptoms of Depression

People who become depressed will experience extreme sadness that is profound and not always related to a traumatic or life-altering event. The already-present depression can worsen however, if such events occur, such as the loss of a loved one, change in careers or moving to a new location, away from friends and family.

Depression also causes a loss of ability to enjoy things that were once pleasurable or to become motivated by things that were previously of interest. Depressed people often have a lack of energy and will feel fatigued and a need to sleep more than the average person not suffering from depression. For thyroid patients, thyroid hormone imbalance can directly cause or contribute to worsening depression.

Adequate Thyroid Treatment

When depression persists in thyroid patients who are being treated, the first and most important thing to consider is whether the treatment is adequate. A person who is diagnosed with hypothyroidism for example and hyperthyroid patients who become hypothyroid after surgical removal or ablation of their thyroid glands (thyroidectomy or radioactive iodine destruction), need to be adequately treated with thyroid hormone replacement therapy. If their dose is not at a level that fully restores their metabolism, they may remain in a state of unresolved symptoms, including those of depression.

Some thyroid specializing doctors and endocrinologists set a goal for TSH of from about 1.0 to 2.0 to start with as mentioned previously. They may increase the dose to suppress TSH further, staying within normal values once adequate time is given to see if satisfactory symptom relief is achieved but is still not occurring. Even small increases in dose can make a difference in how the patient responds to treatment, including improvement in depressed mood. Some doctors will also retest the actual thyroid hormone levels - T4 and T3, in addition to TSH to make sure the levels all correlate properly before considering additional drug or psychiatric treatment therapies.

Other Treatment Options for Depressed Thyroid Patients

As stated previously, research studies of hypothyroid patients have concluded that treatment-resistant depression is better resolved in some patients if a thyroid hormone replacement dose contains "T3 hormone" and not T4 only. There are brands of T3 thyroid hormone available and it is available already combined with T4. A treating doctor may be willing to prescribe a trial of T3 in treated patients who retain depression symptoms if they feel they are proper candidates for it (i.e. they are not hyper-sensitive to oral T3).

When best thyroid hormone treatment options have been tried and depression still persists, patients may need to be prescribed anti-depressant medications or referred for psychiatric therapies. In cases of severe depression, these added options may need to be administered immediately.

A highly successful psychiatric therapy used to treat both anxiety and depression, is one called "Cognitive Behavioral Therapy". A class of antidepressant drugs called Selective Serotonin Reuptake Inhibitors (SSRIs) has also proven to be effective in many cases of depression and/or anxiety conditions. Some patients may find significant symptom-relief from a combination of drug and psychiatric therapies and may respond favorably enough over time, so that they can slowly wean off of one or both treatments, under close supervision of their treating doctor(s).

CHAPTER TWELVE

Sub clinical Hypothyroidism Treatment Challenges

Treating Mild Under active Thyroid Conditions

Sub clinical hypothyroidism is a term meaning an under-active thyroid gland is not at full-blown level (overt) and knowing when to treat these cases can be difficult for doctors.

Some hypothyroid patients experience significant symptoms even when their diagnostic blood labs indicate that their thyroid hormones are only mildly deficient. In these type cases, symptoms should be a consideration in deciding whether or not to begin thyroid hormone replacement therapy as well as determining if the patient has thyroid autoimmunity causing their condition. If auto-antibodies are the cause, starting treatment can help prevent antibodies from further increasing and causing further inflammation in the gland which can contribute to goiter (thyroid gland swelling) and other potential symptoms in the body.

Mild Hypothyroidism Detected by TSH

Most cases of sub clinical hypothyroidism are revealed by an elevated TSH level (Thyroid Stimulating Hormone). This pituitary hormone, coming from the brain-gland that regulates thyroid function, increases to abnormally high levels when thyroid hormones begin to decrease (onset of hypothyroidism). The thyroid hormones, T4 and T3 will at the same time, fall within normal values, although they may be at lower-normal or even borderline-low.

Regardless of where the actual thyroid hormones fall within the normal range, if TSH is elevated even slightly above normal, this usually indicates that the thyroid gland is struggling to produce normal amounts of thyroid hormone to supply the body for maintaining normal metabolism. At this point, most patients do not experience noticeable symptoms, while a small percent of them do experience them and for some, symptoms can be significant. Another factor in whether symptoms are beginning depends on how close a sub clinical case is to becoming full-blown, or what is sometimes referred to as "overt hypothyroidism".

What TSH Level Merits Treating Hypothyroidism?

This question has led to some controversy in medical circles because there are two concerns involved with this issue. One being, that not treating sub clinical cases of hypothyroidism can lead to elevated cholesterol levels, contributing to heart disease over time. The other being, that by treating early, when a patient does not yet fully need replacement thyroid hormone administered, it could induce mild thyrotoxicity (abnormal elevations in thyroid hormones). If treatment does cause mild hyperthyroidism in a patient, it can contribute to osteoporosis and arrhythmias in the heart (abnormal beats).

Some doctors want to see the TSH level elevated to a "10.0" or above before they begin treating hypothyroidism if thyroid hormones continue to stay within normal range. The AACE (American Association of Clinical Endocrinologists) however recently published recommendations in the year 2002, encouraging doctors to consider treating patients whose TSH levels reach levels above "3.04". They also recommended narrowing the diagnostic TSH range to "0.3 to 3.0" which will detect more cases of developing thyroid hormone disorders.

Symptoms and Thyroid Autoimmunity

If a patient with sub clinical hypothyroidism tests positive for thyroid antibodies, this may prompt a doctor to begin treatment due to the fact that thyroid autoimmunity increases the rate of progression to overt hypothyroidism. Some cases of mild under-active thyroid glands are age-related or may have no apparent cause and these can remain in a mild state, not causing symptoms. These cases may not require treatment but will simply need to be monitored closely by blood retests of thyroid levels once or twice yearly.

If symptoms are present in mildly hypothyroid patients, this should be a consideration by doctors monitoring these cases because symptoms can affect quality-of-life in these patients. If additional blood testing reveals elevated cholesterol levels in these patients, this is an important consideration as well because treating with thyroid hormone replacement may be less difficult than treating with cholesterol lowering drugs (statins) which can produce a variety of potential side effects.

CHAPTER THIRTEEN

Best Thyroid Hormone Blood Tests

Diagnostic and Treatment Medical Lab Testing

There are a variety of tests used to both detect thyroid hormone imbalances and to monitor the treatments for them.

Which blood test is best depends on each individual case and depends on factors such as whether the case involves diagnosing thyroid hormone imbalance or if it is follow-up on treatment to correct a problem.

TSH the Most Sensitive Test

Thyroid Stimulating Hormone (TSH) is a pituitary gland hormone as previously mentioned, which is sent from the brain-center or what might be referred to as the "central command post" that monitors and regulates the amount of thyroid hormone released from the thyroid gland. It increases when the thyroid needs to produce more hormone and it decreases when it needs to produce less but in a non-diseased thyroid gland, these fluctuations stay within normal values. When hypothyroidism (under-active thyroid) or hyperthyroidism (overactive thyroid) occurs, TSH will begin to fall outside of the normal values range.

Because of how finely-tuned TSH keeps the thyroid gland, it will change its level in the body with even to most subtle changes in thyroid function. If for example the thyroid becomes less able to provide adequate hormone in the body due to damage in the gland from a disease process affecting it, TSH will increase in level before thyroid hormones decrease in levels. It will continue to increase to higher levels as the thyroid becomes unable to supply normal amounts. During its attempt to keep the thyroid going at normal speed, the TSH hormone will first become mildly abnormal on blood lab tests. This makes TSH the single best and earliest indicator of developing thyroid hormone imbalance that is available.

Free T4 and Free T3

The T3 and T4 thyroid hormone levels can be tested as the "total" levels or as the "free" levels. Many thyroid specialists and endocrinologists believe that the free levels are the better blood tests. This is due to the fact that patients, who are undergoing cortisol steroid treatments for example or estrogen therapy or have certain medical conditions such as liver disease or pregnancy, can experience a change in the level of a thyroid protein called TBG (thyroxine-binding globulin). Much of the T3 is bound in the blood by this protein (total level) with the free, unbound T3 that is left over, being more active in regulating bodily metabolism. This is why some thyroid specialists prefer to test the free unbound levels.

Certain types of scenarios can change the free-circulating level of remaining T3 hormone in the body that is available including cases of thyroid disease. Depending on each particular case, this can result in Total T3 testing normal, while the Free T3 will test outside of normal values, better detecting thyroid hormone imbalances in some cases.

These two thyroid hormones (T3 and T4) are tested both to detect thyroid hormone imbalances and to monitor replacement hormone therapies. They are also sometimes tested to monitor thyroid hormone levels in hyperthyroid patients who have received treatment to slow down abnormally high thyroid hormone production or to retest their levels after they have had their thyroid glands removed as a treatment procedure.

Often, TSH is added to the Free T3 and Free T4 for a more thorough evaluation of patients because TSH alone will not always detect all types of thyroid hormone disorders, such as those caused by a problem within the thyroid-regulating brain glands rather than a problem within the thyroid gland itself.

Thyroid Panels

These groupings of tests, are ordered to better evaluate patients being diagnosed and will include both TSH and thyroid hormone levels (T3 and/or T4). A thyroid panel is often a better diagnostic tool than is TSH alone or a single thyroid hormone level. This is because of factors including those discussed in the previous subheadings in which a thyroid hormone problem can be either primary (within the gland) or secondary (outside of the gland).

This can also be true of thyroid hormone therapies in which TSH alone is not accurate in monitoring treatment due to regulating brain gland problems or due to a problem with only one thyroid hormone level rather than both. The need for varied tests or for more thorough types of thyroid blood tests can occur with "Low T3 Syndromes" or in cases of "impaired conversion of T4 into T3" that is experienced by some thyroid patients taking T4 only replacement hormone medications.

CHAPTER FOURTEEN

Things That Affect Thyroid Hormones in the Body

Facts Treated Thyroid Patients Need to Know

With treated hypothyroidism the therapy is a "set dose" of thyroid hormone replacement. Patients need to be aware of things that can affect thyroid hormone levels in the body.

When a person's own thyroid gland is supplying hormone to the body, the levels will fluctuate as there is a need for them to do so. The pituitary gland in the brain regulates the amount of thyroid hormone released via stimulation of the thyroid gland by Thyroid Stimulating Hormone - TSH.

With thyroid hormone replacement therapy to treat an under active thyroid gland, the dose administered remains steady in the body and does not fluctuate due to things that might change the amount of hormone that is needed. This fact demonstrates the need by treated hypothyroid patients to know what things in their diets and lifestyle practices can affect thyroid hormone levels in the body.

Hard Physical Exercise

While exercise has many benefits, both physical and emotional, hard physical activity can have a lowering affect on thyroid hormone levels. It is important for hypothyroid patients to pace their exercise regimens, so that they do not exceed their tolerance level because thyroid hormones will not rise to meet the extra demand when a set-dose is being taken. The resulting effect can be severe fatigue and slow recovery from hard physical activity. Exercise should be built upon slowly to a reasonable level and afterward maintained at the proper level, so that a thyroid hormone dose remains adequate, reflected in follow up blood retests that monitor the dose.

Alcohol, Caffeine and Smoking

Medical research studies have shown that alcohol consumption can negatively affect thyroid hormone levels and is especially true in pregnant women who can cause thyroid function to drop in both their own bodies and that of their fetuses with alcohol use. Alcohol acts as both a stimulant and a depressant and it could be that there are increases in thyroid hormones with alcohol use in smaller amounts that are followed by decreases in the levels with increased or prolonged alcohol use.

Another stimulant that has been shown to alter thyroid hormone production, is caffeine and medical studies done with animal models have shown that caffeine consumption temporarily increases thyroid hormone levels, which might cause a temporary increase in energy as well but as with any stimulant, will also cause a resulting crash when levels drop back down to normal levels. Hypothyroid patients feel these fluctuations more intensely than do people with normal thyroid function whose bodies can adjust the thyroid hormone levels in response to these type influences.

A third stimulant that has also been studied by medical research groups but in this case using human models, is tobacco smoking. Studies have shown that smokers have elevated thyroid hormone levels and decreased TSH levels. Some of the conclusions in these studies state that smokers have a three-fold increased risk for developing Graves' disease, the autoimmune-cause of hyperthyroidism (overactive).

In hypothyroid patients with Hashimoto's thyroiditis (autoimmune cause), smoking may place them at higher risk for episodes of Hashitoxicosis (hyperthyroid phases) or for transitioning over to Graves' disease. A substantial risk that has been confirmed in medical research is the fact that smoking increases chances for the development of "Thyroid Eye Disease" (inflammatory condition) in autoimmune thyroid disorder patients.

Goitrogen Foods

It is a well known fact that eating foods high in calcium and/or iron or taking supplements containing these elements can hinder absorption of a thyroid hormone dose, unless taken at least four hours apart from the dose (some sources recommend six hours). There are, however other foods that can actually cause thyroid hormone levels to decrease, regardless of when eaten, called "goitrogens". These type foods are medically recognized for their ability to lower thyroid hormone levels in the body due to their effect in blocking the action of "thyroid peroxidase" (protein/enzyme).

One major food group well-known for its thyroid hormone diminishing ability is soy products. Reading ingredient labels can reveal which products contain soy apart from the obvious ones. Other foods that can have a goitrogenic affect are those from the cruciferous family of vegetables.

These include:

• mustard

• rutabaga

• turnips

• broccoli

• brussel sprouts

• cabbage

• cauliflower

• kale

• kohlrabi

• spinach

• radishes

Nuts, grains and fruits in the goitrogen category include the following:

• millet

• peanuts

• soybeans

• strawberries

• peaches

Treated hypothyroid patients should avoid these foods beyond small servings (large portions) and thoroughly cooking them can help diminish their goitrogenic effects.

CHAPTER FIFTEEN

Thyroid Symptoms May Need Special Attention

When Hormone Replacement Does Not Give Adequate Symptom Relief

While most symptoms are relieved with treatments designed for thyroid hormone imbalances there are some common problem-symptoms that treated patients commonly experience.

The symptoms addressed in this article can also be those that require additional attention by the patient and/or the treating doctor, if thyroid treatment alone does not satisfactorily alleviate them.

Fatigue

This symptom often not relieved satisfactorily in treated thyroid patients may be the number one problem affecting them, according to some surveys. It is also a strong possibility that fatigue is associated with thyroid autoimmunity (the disease process) and not a result of abnormal thyroid hormone levels alone. In addition to Fibromyalgia being commonly suspected in thyroid patients before they receive definitive diagnoses of thyroid problems, they are also commonly suspected of having Chronic Fatigue Syndrome (CFS) before proper blood testing reveals thyroid hormone abnormalities. Some patients after being well-treated and that have had all other possible causes of fatigue ruled-out, may receive a diagnosis of CFS being co-morbid (co-occurring) with thyroid disease.

The U.S. Centers for Disease Control now recognizes the fact that thyroid disease can co-exist with CFS and other medical studies conclude that autoimmune diseases of any kind may serve as a trigger for causing CFS. Things that can help patients who continue experiencing fatigue despite proper thyroid treatment, would include supplementing with Vitamins B5, B5, B6, B12, C and E, folic acid, CoQ10 and the herbal remedies called ginkgo biloba and ginseng. These supplements have been found to increase cellular energy in the body and may help to increase oxygen levels in the blood.

A patient should inform their doctor when taking any new supplements of any kind, as a precaution against their contraindicating (reacting adversely) with other treatments being administered.

Weight Gain and Difficulty Losing

This problem symptom may be one of the most concerning and is probably second only to unrelieved fatigue. Weight gain is a very frustrating symptom and one thyroid patients have strong desire to see corrected through their treatments. This problem is more common in hypothyroid patients because hyperthyroidism typically causes weight loss rather than weight gain. Hyperthyroid patients however, do become hypothyroid if their case requires thyroid removal by surgical thyroidectomy or radioactive iodine ablation. It typically requires extra effort for treated hypothyroid patients to lose weight and to control it.

It is very important that hypothyroidism is adequately treated because under-treatment can contribute to weight problems from slowed metabolism and body fluid retention (myxedema). There are many diet plans available however; the keys to weight loss and control include the following.

• reducing calorie intake (i.e. simple carbohydrates: candies, pies, cookies and soft drinks)

• eating healthy foods (i.e. fruits, vegetables, nuts and grains)

• eliminating refined sugars as much as possible

• regular exercise

The claims of magical diets or ones that take no effort are usually false and weight loss remedies containing stimulants can be unhealthy and dangerous in some cases.

Joint and Muscle Aches

Many hypothyroid patients report that their first symptoms of thyroid disease were rheumatic ones, meaning joint and muscle aches and stiffness. Some patients in fact were believed to be experiencing Fibromyalgia Syndrome before receiving definitive diagnoses of thyroid disorders. Unfortunately some patients retain a degree of rheumatic symptoms even when well-treated. According the medical research studies, this can be due to "thyroid autoimmunity", meaning thyroid disease caused by auto-antibodies. These thyroid antibodies cause a degree of inflammation in the body which can settle in muscles and joints, causing mild to moderate aches and stiffness.

If rheumatic symptoms are severe and there is swelling or redness around joints, tests to detect or rule out Rheumatoid Arthritis (RA) should be conducted. Autoimmune thyroid diseases place patients at higher risk for other autoimmune conditions, including RA. When these type symptoms are thyroid-related, making sure replacement hormone therapy is at the proper level is important and some medical research has shown that supplementing with the mineral selenium may also help lower auto-antibody activity. Over-the-counter anti-inflammatory drugs can also help reduce symptoms but these and any other drugs or supplements, should be approved by the patient's treating doctor, as a precaution against their interfering with other treatments currently being administered.

Emotional Symptoms

This area of symptomology is also common in both hypothyroid and hyperthyroid disorders as addressed in a previous chapter. Anxiety and/or depression can result from either type of thyroid hormone imbalance but medical research has also shown that emotional disorders can be associated with the disease process itself (thyroid autoimmunity). Most cases of hypothyroidism in industrialized countries are caused by "Hashimoto's thyroiditis" and most cases of hyperthyroidism are caused by Graves' disease. These are the autoimmune diseases that are the root cause. Medical research studies have concluded that the auto-antibodies that characterize these diseases may be responsible for emotional symptoms and disorders rather than abnormal hormone levels alone.

Patients with unresolved emotional disorder symptoms may need the added benefit of psychiatric therapies such as Cognitive Behavioral Therapy and/or psychotropic medications. Prescription-medications that can help reduce anxiety and stress symptoms, include the following.

• benzodiazepines (i.e. Xanax)

• adrenergic receptor antagonists (i.e. Buspirone).

• daily regimen antidepressants - SSRI drugs (i.e. Paxil, Prozac, Zoloft)

Natural supplements that have been reported to help relieve anxiety and depression symptoms include the following.

• Bach's Rescue Remedy

• Panicyl

- St. John's Wort

- Valerian extract

- GABA

- SAMe

- Passion Flower

Any non-prescription supplements a patient may take need to be reported to their doctor to make sure he finds no risks of adverse reactions by adding them to medical treatments that are already being administered.

CHAPTER SIXTEEN

Treated Hypothyroidism and Fatigue

When Tiredness does Not Resolve with Thyroid Treatment

Feeling tired and fatigued is common in treated hypothyroid patients as addressed in a previous chapter. Surveys of treated patients have shown it to be one of the most common unresolved symptoms they experience. This chapter will be dedicated to further addressing this concerning and sometimes stubborn symptom.

When hypothyroid patients feel lack of energy or even totally exhausted despite being treated for hypothyroidism, there are several areas to consider, that might hold an answer to this lingering problem.

Optimized Thyroid Hormone Replacement

The first thing to consider when a patient continues to feel tired after being treated for hypothyroidism is whether or not their thyroid hormone therapy is at optimal or sub-optimal levels. Patients often have a narrow treatment range where the best symptom relief can be found or what might be referred to as their "set-point" as mentioned in an earlier chapter. This is that optimal level of thyroid hormone dose that best relieves their symptoms of hypothyroidism.

If for example, a patient has been treated to get their T4 and T3 thyroid hormone levels at approximately mid-range or only slightly above and their TSH level is still above lower-normal, this would suggest that a dose increase can be administered by the treating doctor in attempt toward better symptom-relief. This might be referred to as "wiggle room" to safely tweak the dose for better results.

TSH is suppressed with a thyroid hormone dose when it is elevated due to hypothyroidism. If for example, lowest normal at the blood lab used to monitor a hypothyroid patient's hormone therapy is "0.05" (a half-point) but their TSH has only been suppressed down to about 3.0 (three points), a trial of a dose to suppress it further down to about 1.0 should not place them at risk for over treatment (dose induced thyrotoxicity). If T4 and T3 levels stay within higher-normal range at this TSH level, this too would be reassurance against over-treatment and might also yield a much better level of symptom-relief for fatigue.

Thorough Blood Lab Evaluation

Hypothyroid patients are at higher risk for other problems, such as anemia, including the type caused by low vitamin B12 levels, celiac disease (intolerance to gluten in the diet), diabetes and problems with adrenal and sex hormone levels. If fatigue or other symptoms continue in a hypothyroid patient who is well-treated and whose blood lab retests show that their thyroid hormone therapy dose has been optimized, thorough blood testing for these other disorders would be merited.

Each of these disorders can be detected or ruled out via diagnostic blood lab testing. In addition to complete blood counts, glucose levels, Vitamin B12, other hormone levels (i.e. sex and adrenal) and tests for antibodies that reveal Celiac disease (gluten-sensitive enteropathy), patients should also be tested for systemic autoimmunity via the ANA blood test and for systemic inflammation via the ESR blood test. These latter mentioned two tests can help to rule out or confirm other inflammatory and autoimmune diseases that may be present in the body, such as Lupus and Rheumatoid Arthritis, each of which can present with fatigue as a major symptom.

Thyroid Autoimmunity Contributes to Fatigue

While it is not often noted in medical studies or by doctors when communicating with their patients, "thyroid autoimmunity" (Hashimoto's thyroiditis) which is the most common cause of hypothyroidism in industrialized countries can also contribute to symptoms apart from corrected thyroid hormone levels.

Studies published on PubMed-U.S. National Institutes of Health - medical research website, state that thyroid autoimmunity (antibodies) can contribute to symptom manifestations ranging from rheumatic ones (joint and muscle problems) to severe life-threatening conditions such as Hashimoto's Ecephalopathy (rare inflammatory response in the brain). This can be true despite having abnormal thyroid hormone levels well-treated and corrected to optimal levels. Thyroid autoimmunity for example, is an inflammatory condition that can cause goiter as a first symptom, before thyroid hormone levels fall out of the normal range.

Supplements and Methods that can help Fatigue

When treatment for hypothyroidism has been optimized and other co-existing problems addressed or ruled out, additional steps can be taken to help with unrelieved fatigue. Natural supplements that can help energy levels include B vitamins, such as B-5, B-6 and B-12. There are sublingual brands of B-12 available (liquid for under the tongue) that can help maintain energy by dosing two to three times a day as needed. Many brands of B12 are formulated with Vitamin C added to help with absorption and are a combination that is helpful for healthy adrenal gland function as well.

Other natural supplements (not exceeded at manufacturer's recommended dose) that can help with fatigue include:

• coenzyme Q10

• folic acid

• thiamine

• niacin

• tyrosine

The effectiveness of some nutrients and vitamins do however also depend upon a healthy diet to work well in the body. It bears repeating that eliminating refined sugars and stimulants like caffeine and alcohol and eating plenty of fruits, vegetables, nuts and grains can be helpful. Limiting any intake of goitrogen foods (listed previously) that have a lowering effect on thyroid hormones can also help. These foods are more problem-some if not fully cooked or not eaten in small, infrequent servings. To also mention again - exercise in moderation often helps with energy levels but should only be done at tolerance-level or can otherwise exacerbate fatigue levels.

If fatigue is chronic and all other causes have been eliminated, a diagnosis of Chronic Fatigue Syndrome might result. Both CFS and Fibromyalgia have been found to affect thyroid patients more commonly than the general public.

CHAPTER SEVENTEEN

Qualities Needed in Hypothyroid Treating Doctors

What to Look for in Thyroid Specialists

The symptoms of hypothyroidism can be concerning and severe to a thyroid patient. This, points to the great importance in a qualified hypothyroid treatment specialist.

People needing treatment for hypothyroidism should seek doctors who are qualified in optimizing thyroid hormone therapy the best possible for each of their patients but who also monitor their patients for potential co-morbid conditions and treatment complications.

Palpation for Goiter and Thyroid Nodules

The vast majority of hypothyroid patients have the condition due to diseased thyroid glands. Thyroid specializing doctors should check their new patients for goiter (thyroid gland swelling) and for thyroid nodules (tumorous growths) by palpation. This means the doctor uses fingertips to feel for growths within the thyroid gland that might merit further investigation if found.

Most thyroid nodules are not suspicious for being malignant (cancerous) but if one is found that is of significant size or that is singular and of a solid-texture (solid, cold nodule) rather than among a group of nodules (multi-nodular), additional testing would likely be ordered for further evaluation. These would be precautionary measures, to rule out the possibility of thyroid cancer and the risk for obstructed breathing and/or swallowing if goiters or nodules of significant size are found or those that pose a danger of growing larger.

Diagnostic Blood Testing

Thyroid specializing doctors should not limit diagnosis of thyroid disorders to the TSH blood test only. He or she should also not limit the monitoring of thyroid hormone replacement therapy with the TSH level alone. Some thyroid hormone disorders may present with normal TSH levels such as certain types of secondary hypothyroidism. This includes cases of Central Hypothyroidism when TSH may test at normal values, low-normal or even below normal, with thyroid hormone levels (T4 and T3) also at below normal. TSH is supposed to elevate with hypothyroidism but fails to do so in these cases. The failure of TSH to rise can be due to a problem in the pituitary, the brain-gland that regulates thyroid function.

Thorough Monitoring of Newly-Treated Hypothyroid Patients

While TSH is accurate in monitoring thyroid hormone therapy in most cases, if central Hypothyroidism is being treated, the T4 and/or T3 thyroid hormones will also need to be tested. It is also a reasonable precaution to test thyroid hormone levels in addition to TSH in all newly-treated hypothyroid patients for at least the first couple of follow-up blood retests, to make sure both T4 and T3 are staying at proper levels and are correlating properly with TSH. Once it is determined that TSH is all that is needed to monitor a patient's treatment, the doctor can at that time switch to using it as the only test.

Newly treated hypothyroid patients should be blood retested at no longer than 3-month intervals, while patients who are stable on a dose of replacement thyroid hormone that has reached optimal level, may only need retested once every 6-months. A treating doctor should also instruct their patients to report any symptoms that may appear between blood retests that might indicate either over-treatment (hyperthyroid) or under-treatment (hypothyroid) and the possible need for a dose adjustment.

Adjusting Thyroid Hormone Replacement Doses

Some thyroid doctors have targeted treatment goals rather than simply treating hypothyroid patients on replacement hormone doses to get their levels anywhere within normal values. However, less than mid-range normal values for the

T4 and T3 or low-normal values may keep some patients in a state of unrelieved hypothyroid symptoms.

Doctors who are more targeted to achieve best results for their hypothyroid patients will be willing to adjust their doses of hormone therapy to reach at least mid-range or higher-normal T4 and T3 levels. This may require suppressing the TSH to very low-normal readings in some patients and will require that the treating doctor is willing to make the needed dose adjustments to reach the target therapy goal.

Some patients may see more symptom relief with a different type of prescription thyroid hormone (T4 only or combination T4/T3) or a different brand (synthetic or natural) and a doctor should be willing to switch patients to a trial of another type if the initial brand they started treatment with yields unsatisfactory results.

SECTION TWO: **Everything about Hyperthyroidism**

CHAPTER ONE

Hyperthyroidism Basic Facts

Overactive Thyroid Gland General Information

Hyperthyroid disorders account for approximately 20% of thyroid disorder cases. An overactive thyroid gland can cause an array of symptoms but treatments are available.

Hyperthyroidism is a term meaning a person's bodily metabolism is abnormally sped up due to the T3 and/or T4 thyroid hormone levels increasing too high in the body. Symptoms vary in severity among individuals, according to how advanced hyperthyroidism has become at the time of diagnosis.

Major Causes of Hyperthyroidism

Most cases of hyperthyroidism are caused by Graves' disease, the autoimmune disease of the thyroid gland in which auto-antibodies sent from the immune system cause stimulation of excessive amounts of thyroid hormone production. Graves' patients experience thyroid gland inflammation and enlargement to varied degrees, referred to as "toxic diffuse goiters". Thyroid autoimmunity is a "primary" cause of an overactive thyroid gland.

Another primary cause of an overactive thyroid gland would include "hot nodules", which are tumorous-growths in the gland that absorb iodine in the body and begin producing thyroid hormone just as normal thyroid tissue does.

Less common "secondary" causes of hyperthyroidism include excessive intake of iodine which can also act as a trigger for primary thyroid autoimmunity. Temporary types, of thyroiditis occurring in pregnant women or following giving birth or as a result of viral illnesses that settle in the thyroid gland, will cause a short-term phase of hyperthyroidism. Treated hypothyroid patients can become hyperthyroid from taking too high a dose of thyroid hormone replacement, sometimes referred to as "dose induced thyrotoxicity".

Hyperthyroid Symptoms

The symptoms of a sped up metabolism from hyperthyroidism include:

• nervousness and anxiety

• tremor (especially in the hands)

• rapid pulse and breathing

• hypertension

• diarrhea

• oily skin and hair

• increased sweating

• increased hunger and thirst

• changes in menstrual cycle and sex drive

• goiter

• rapid weight loss

Patients with Graves' disease may also experience symptoms of muscle weakness and wasting referred to as "myopathy". They may also develop an inflammatory condition affecting the eyes called "Graves' Ophthalmopathy" or "Thyroid Eye Disease".

Diagnosis

Blood tests of thyroid hormone levels and/or the TSH level can help to diagnose hyperthyroidism. Thyroid hormones (T4 and T3) will elevate to levels above normal values, while TSH (pituitary hormone) will decrease to levels below normal values. When testing is conducted to determine the cause of hyperthyroidism, blood tests for thyroid antibodies may be ordered to confirm or rule out Graves' disease as the cause.

A Radioactive Iodine Uptake Test (RAIU) might also be performed to determine if the thyroid gland is absorbing high levels of iodine which can indicate that it is overactive. If only a certain area of the gland is absorbing high levels of iodine, this can point to hot nodules and an additional Radioactive Iodine Scan (radiology camera) might also be performed at the same time or separately to further evaluate nodules in the gland.

Treatment

In some cases of hyperthyroidism, the administering of anti-thyroid drugs designed to slow thyroid hormone production will be the initial treatment and possible the only one needed. Beta-blocker medications that moderate the activity of adrenaline in the body can help to alleviate symptoms and may be combined with anti-thyroid drugs.

Surgical procedures are required in some cases of hot nodules, to remove them or part of the thyroid gland if multi-nodules are present (several). Thyroid removal surgery called "thyroidectomy" may also be needed in cases of Graves' disease that cannot be controlled by drug therapies or the gland may be ablated (destroyed) through administering radioactive iodine in a large enough to dose to kill-out the entire gland.

Afterward, patients whose thyroid glands are ablated or removed will require thyroid hormone replacement to treat resulting hypothyroidism, as a lifelong treatment.

CHAPTER TWO

Major Causes of Hyperthyroidism and Treatments

Common Contributors to Thyrotoxicity

As mentioned previously, approximately 20% of thyroid disease cases are hyperthyroid conditions. There are several causes for overactive thyroid disorders and treatments available for them.

The term "thyrotoxicity" simply means that abnormally high levels of thyroid hormone in the body are causing a toxic reaction also referred to as "hyperthyroidism". While the majority of hyperthyroid conditions are a result of auto-antibodies that stimulate excessive thyroid hormone levels, there are a number of other causes as addressed in the subheadings that follow.

Temporary Thyroiditis

Some people experiencing viral infections or pregnancies will have a resulting inflammatory reaction in their thyroid glands called "thyroiditis". Some cases manifest with a painful thyroid gland (sub-acute) while others do not (silent) but the majority of temporary thyroiditis conditions start with a phase of hyperthyroidism. Treatment for high levels of thyroid hormone is usually not necessary since the condition will resolve on its own over several weeks period of time. Treatment may only require bed rest and anti-inflammatory drugs for fever and thyroid inflammation.

Over-consumption of Iodine

People taking drugs that contain high-iodine content or who consume an excessive amount of iodine-rich foods such as kelp (seaweed) or supplements that contain higher-than-recommended daily allowances of iodine can cause hyperthyroidism to be induced. In these cases, if the excessive iodine intake does not trigger an autoimmune response, causing permanent hyperthyroidism, the treatment would simply be to discontinue use of the products containing high levels of iodine.

Hot Nodules

Thyroid nodules are tumor-like growths that can develop within the thyroid gland. The majority of them do not affect thyroid hormone levels but a small percent can present as "hot nodules". This means the nodule has taken on features similar to thyroid gland tissue and is absorbing iodine coming into the body and producing thyroid hormones from it. This adds more thyroid hormone production to what the gland is already normally producing, causing the levels to become abnormally high.

Treatment for hot nodules may include surgical removal of them or removal of part of the thyroid gland (partial or sub-total thyroidectomy or lobectomy) or of the entire gland (total thyroidectomy). Once thyroid tissue is removed via a corrective procedure, thyroid hormone replacement may also become necessary afterward, as a life long treatment.

Over-treated Hypothyroidism

Thyroid hormone replacement therapy is administered by an oral dose of T4 or combination T4 and T3 prescription thyroid hormone medication. The dose is then monitored through follow-up blood retests of the hormone levels in the patient's body. If a dose is too high and over-replacement is occurring, medication-induced thyrotoxicity can occur. The treatment would be to reduce the patient's dose and to possibly stop the dose temporarily so that their thyroid hormone levels decrease back down into the normal values range. Afterward the corrected dose-level would also need to be monitored via blood retests and at reasonable intervals throughout the patient's life.

Thyroid Autoimmunity

Graves' disease is the autoimmune cause of progressive hyperthyroidism in which auto-antibodies stimulate excessive production of thyroid hormones. Hashitoxicosis is also an autoimmune cause of hyperthyroidism but in this case, patients with Hashimoto's thyroiditis that typically causes progressive hypothyroidism (under-active) will first see the condition manifest with a phase of temporary hyperthyroidism.

Most patients experiencing Hashitoxicosis will not have additional flares of the condition once it initially resolves, although some do experience milder fluctuations in thyroid hormones due to flares of thyroiditis (phases of increased inflammation). In rare cases, Hashimoto's thyroiditis will transition over to Graves' disease but most patients remain hypothyroid and require life-long thyroid hormone replacement therapy.

Treatment for cases of hyperthyroidism from Graves' disease may include anti-thyroid drugs to reduce elevated thyroid hormone levels, beta-blocker medications to reduce hyperthyroid symptoms and possible eventual thyroid removal by surgery (thyroidectomy) or destruction of the gland by radioactive iodine (ablation).

CHAPTER THREE

Graves' Disease Hyperthyroidism and Treatments

Autoimmune Caused Hyperthyroidism

As mentioned in a previous chapter, Graves' disease is the leading cause of hyperthyroidism. Complications can include hypertension, cardiac arrhythmias and thyroid eye disease but treatments are available.

Graves' disease is an autoimmune condition affecting the thyroid gland that results in abnormally high levels of thyroid hormone to be released into the body causing hyperthyroidism. There is no cure for Graves' but progression of the disease can be halted by removing the thyroid gland. Mild to moderate cases may be successfully treated through drug therapies.

How Common is Graves' Disease?

Graves' disease affects up to 1% of the U.S. population or up to 3-million people, which is about 5 in every 10,000 people and is 7 times more common in women than in men. Graves' patients are among the 190 million people worldwide who experience goiters but in the case of Graves' the goiter is "toxic" (toxic diffuse goiter), meaning it is causing abnormally high thyroid hormone levels or "thyrotoxicity" (hyperthyroidism).

Graves' patients can experience complications from the disease, including an inflammatory condition in the eyes called "Thyroid Eye Disease" or "Graves' Ophthalmology". It is estimated that about half (50%) of all Graves' patient will develop this complication of the disease affecting the eyes.

Is Hyperthyroidism Present in all Graves' Patients?

The point at which hyperthyroidism sets in varies among those found to have the auto-antibodies causing Graves' disease, called "Thyroid Stimulating Immunglobulin" (TSI). Most patients may be positive for these "thyroid antibodies" months or years before the level of them becomes elevated enough to cause hyperthyroidism. The reason this may be the case is due to the fact that most people who are found to have Graves', are tested because they are already manifesting the signs or symptoms of hyperthyroidism. There are cases in which Graves' patients experience mild, early-onset goiters before their thyroid hormone levels become abnormally high.

Thyroid Antibodies common to both Graves' and Hashimoto's

The TSI are not the only antibodies present with Graves' but will co-exist with other thyroid antibodies that cause thyroid cell destruction, including the anti-thyroidperoxidase (Anti-TPO) and/or the anti-thyroglobulin (Anti-TG). These latter two mentioned antibodies are also present in Hashimoto's thyroiditis (autoimmune hypothyroidism) patients but are usually found in lower titers (positive lab measurements) in Graves' patients.

Some Hashimoto's patients in fact are also found to be positive for TSI antibodies that typically cause Graves' but are in lower titers and may cause temporary hyperthyroid phases (Hashitoxicosis). These facts demonstrate how closely related these two autoimmune thyroid diseases are. It also offers explanation as to why some Graves' patients transition to Hashimoto's over time and the reverse has also been know to happen, although not common.

Symptoms and Treatment for Graves' Hyperthyroidism

When thyroid hormone levels have become abnormally high, causing the body's metabolism to become sped up, hyperthyroidism symptoms will develop. These include increased energy, nervousness and anxiety, rapid heart rate, hypertension, excessive sweating, diarrhea and weight loss. If Thyroid Eye Disease develops, the additional symptoms may include bulging, dryness, double vision (diplopia), and irritation of the eyeballs.

Some cases of Graves'-caused hyperthyroidism are successfully treated with anti-thyroid drugs, which block thyroid hormone, reducing the amount entering the cells of the body and/or beta-blockers, which block the effects of epinephrine (adrenaline). When epinephrine is elevated in the body, it can cause cardiac arrhythmias and hypertension and elevated thyroid hormone levels speed up all bodily functions as a whole.

Determining which drug is needed or if a combination of them is needed, depends on how severe the hyperthyroidism is. Severe cases of Graves' hyperthyroidism that cannot be successfully treated with drug therapies may require surgical removal of the gland (thyroidectomy) or destruction of the gland using radioactive iodine (ablation). Afterward, patients will need thyroid hormone levels corrected with replacement therapy.

Treatment for Graves' Ophthalmology (Thyroid Eye Disease)

Thyroid Eye Disease (TED) is often treated using anti-inflammatory steroids (corticosteroids) to reduce inflammation, such as Prednisone. Eye drops may also be prescribed to keep dry eyes moistened. In cases when the disease is causing significant pressure on the optic nerve and presents the danger of vision loss, eye surgeries called "orbital radiotherapy" and/or "orbital decompression" may be necessary.

If eye protrusion is causing inability for a patient to close their eyes, surgery may be required to lengthen their eyelids. Many cases of TED have duration of from several months up to about 3 years and will improve spontaneously or with the aid of treatment depending on the severity.

Studies of TED have shown that Graves' patients who smoke more often experience TED or cases that are more severe.

CHAPTER FOUR

Radioactive Iodine Ablation of the Thyroid

Cell Destruction of Diseased Glands

This procedure abbreviated - RAI is performed by giving a patient an oral dose of radioactive iodine, which causes thyroid tissue death to cease its hyper-functioning.

RAI is the most commonly performed treatment for resolving cases of severe hyperthyroidism. Most people with Graves' disease, the most common cause of an overactive thyroid, are recommended for this procedure if medications fail to sufficiently slow-down an over-producing gland.

Patients with papillary or follicular thyroid cancer may also be referred for this procedure, following surgical removal of their glands (total thyroidectomy), to eradicate any remaining thyroid cells that can potentially contain malignancy.

How Does RAI Work?

The goal of RAI includes the following desired results:

• to destroy and eradicate all thyroid tissue and/or malignant cells in the body

• to stop the natural thyroid hormone production in the gland

• to correct hyperthyroidism

• to restore normal metabolism to the body

Once a dose of radioactive iodine that is large enough to completely kill the cells in a thyroid gland has been administered, the iodine is immediately absorbed by the gland. It does this because the thyroid is dependent on iodine to manufacture thyroid hormone. Once iodine enters the body through a person's diet or by oral dosing, the gland absorbs it to regulate bodily metabolism via these hormones.

An overactive thyroid gland will absorb more iodine than a normal-functioning gland will. Patients scheduled for RAI are placed on a "no iodine diet" for two weeks or more previous to the procedure, so that the thyroid gland absorbs the radioactive iodine as completely as possible.

What is the Result?

The radioactivity in the iodine enters the cells of the gland and causes them to die. The goal of the treatment is to fully eradicate all thyroid tissue from the body, so that it ceases to produce thyroid hormone. This will correct the hyperthyroidism.

Once thyroid hormone levels begin falling to lower levels following RAI, the overactive bodily metabolism slows down from the hyperthyroid state. Several weeks following the procedure the patient's thyroid hormone levels will fall to hypothyroid levels (under-active). The resulting hypothyroidism must then be treated (usually lifelong) with

77

thyroid hormone replacement therapy to raise bodily metabolism back to a normal level.

What are the Risks?

RAI is a safe and effective procedure in most cases; there are, however, some medical sources that state that the treatment places some patients at risk for a worsening of thyroid eye disease (inflammatory condition in the eyeballs).

Other side effects that are temporary may include the following:

• sore throat

• dry mouth

• mild nausea

• dizziness

• fatigue

Some patients will rarely also see thyroid tissue that is not fully eradicated from the body that regrows and becomes revitalized and begins producing thyroid hormone. If it does so at an abnormally high level as it did before the procedure, this may require that the treatment be re-administered.

Patients are also required to be quarantined from family and pets for five to seven days due to risk of exposing them to radiation that remains in the body for a period following the procedure and can be spread by close contact.

Some thyroid-treating doctors offer a choice between thyroidectomy and RAI procedures to some of patients in need of thyroid ablation/removal (depending on individual cases). Patients should become educated about both options and fully discuss them with their treating doctor so that they feel comfortable and confident about the procedure they choose to have their doctors perform.

CHAPTER FIVE

Treatment for Hashitoxicosis versus Graves' Disease

Patients with Temporary Hyperthyroidism

When Hashimoto's patients developing hypothyroidism, an under-active thyroid gland, go through "Hashitoxicosis", meaning temporary hyperthyroidism (overactive) they usually only register a slight difference in blood labs or only a mild indication of hyperthyroidism on them due to progressive hypothyroidism trying to take over. In other words, though these patients alternate between hyperthyroidism and hypothyroidism, it is temporary so that lab results of their thyroid hormone levels can at times be neutral or show only mild hyperthyroidism.

These patients may however test positive for "thyroid stimulating immunoglobulin" (TSI), the auto-antibody that typically contributes to Graves' disease (autoimmune hyperthyroidism). Once hypothyroidism does take over, they will need thyroid hormone replacement as a lifelong treatment. With Graves' disease, it settles in long enough to register as full blown hyperthyroidism on blood lab tests of thyroid hormone levels. This plus a high elevation of TSI antibodies can point to a definitive diagnosis of Graves' disease.

Rarely, Hashimoto's and Graves' can co-exist somewhat equally in a thyroid patient, so that they don't fully transition over to one or the other and when this occurs, the treatment may be destruction or surgical removal of the thyroid. Some countries treat these type patients that waver back and forth between the two disease, with a treatment called "block and replace" in which thyroid hormone blocking drugs (anti-thyroid) are first administered, followed by thyroid hormone replacement, once hypothyroidism has been fully induced. This treatment is rarely used in the USA.

Some doctors try an anti-thyroid drug or what's called a "PTU" (propylthiouracil and Carbimazole) that slows thyroid hormone production for Graves'-hyperthyroidism and after a trial of it, will wean the patient off of it after a few months and see if the hyperthyroidism resolves. If not, they will then opt for RAI ablation (Radio Active Iodine destruction of the thyroid gland) or a thyroidectomy (surgical removal). Many will first try a beta-blocker to see if it controls the hyperthyroid symptoms before going on to a PTU or a combination of the two.

If you are recommended for getting a thyroidectomy Vs RAI ask your doctor to go over the procedure with you (risks etc...), or to refer you to a doctor who can, so you can weigh the two options. You might also ask him about anti-thyroid medications if he feels they are another possible option in your case. In short, I would say overt hyperthyroidism on blood lab test results definitely points to Graves' disease. It is not that unusual for offspring of autoimmune thyroid disease parents to develop one or the other because the two diseases (Hashimoto's thyroiditis and Graves' disease) are more closely related than most people realize.

CHAPTER SIX

Why Doctors Sometimes Delay Treatment for Hashimoto's Thyroiditis

Problems with Hashitoxicosis

I created the article following below, from a response I wrote to a fellow thyroid patient experiencing severe anxiety symptoms with their Hashimoto's thyroiditis. I commented on this aspect of their thyroid disease case in the reply that follows.

My Reply:

Sometimes doctors are cautious about starting treatment due to the fact that if they treat when your thyroid hormones are fluctuating upward, which can happen earlier into the onset of Hashimoto's, they could cause you thyrotoxicity (hyperthyroidism). This would make anxiety symptoms even worse. This fluctuation back and forth between hyper (overactive) and hypo (under-active) thyroid levels is common with autoimmune thyroiditis. When hyperthyroid phases are severe, it's called "Hashitoxicosis", so in my opinion, the doctor is wise in monitoring your case a while longer before starting you on thyroid hormone replacement. He likely will be blood retesting your levels at about 3-month intervals or so.

As far as treatment for anxiety symptoms, mine too were severe early into the onset of Hashimoto's thyroiditis and I personally used as-needed anti-anxiety drugs (like Xanax) but I did not use them for longer than a couple of months at a time and usually took half-doses rather than full ones. These type drugs (benzodiazepines) can be addictive and is why they should be taken with some caution. This is just an added option I would mention.

Also, you are absolutely right in that research studies state that Hashimoto's thyroiditis causes anxiety symptoms but strangely there are doctors who do not have knowledge of that fact and will tell patients that the anxiety is not thyroid-related. In addition to medical studies, thousands of patients on forums, message boards and blogs attesting to having anxiety symptoms with Hashimoto's can't all be wrong!

This is just lay-opinion but I would try low dose, as-needed anti-anxiety meds before accepting a prescription for the permanent daily-dosing type, such as SSRI antidepressants. There's nothing wrong with these and they can be greatly helpful when needed but your thyroiditis flares causing anxiety may diminish over a few months or even within a few weeks time, so starting a permanent regimen drug might be an over-kill so-to-speak at this point of observing your case. Certainly if emotional symptoms are severe or overwhelming and an as-needed drug is not helping enough, therapy can be very beneficial, as can permanent type drugs. I would never discourage any of these things when they are proven to be necessary.

CHAPTER SEVEN

Manifestations of Thyroid Eye Disease

Autoimmune Eyeball Problems and Their Treatments

Thyroid Eye Disease more commonly affects people with hyperthyroid conditions but can also occur in hypothyroid patients with thyroid autoimmunity.

Both inflammation and build up of fluid around the eyes can cause them to protrude (exophthalmos) and have an exaggeratedly wide-open appearance with Thyroid Eye Disease (TED), also referred to as "thyroid orbitopathy". The eyeball can also move forward from its position within the eye socket which can become severe in some cases (proptosis).

Patients with TED can experience dryness, redness and irritation within their eyes. A feeling of pressure and grittiness in the eyes can also occur, as well as difficulty with fully closing the eyelids. Treatments are available for this condition associated with cases of thyroid autoimmunity (diseases caused by thyroid antibodies).

Graves' Ophthalmopathy

Medical sources state that Graves' Ophthalmopathy is clinically apparent to varied degrees in up to 50% of Graves' disease patients, although other medical sources state that up to 80% of Graves' patients experience some type of eye symptoms as listed previously. While Graves' is the autoimmune cause of thyrotoxicity, also referred to as "hyperthyroidism" TED can occur in approximately 10% of patients with the auto-antibodies that cause Grave's but whose thyroid hormone levels are euthyroid, meaning within normal values. Only about 2% of Hashimoto's thyroiditis patients (those with autoimmune hypothyroidism) are affected by TED.

Optic Neuropathy

The optic nerves in the eyes of TED patients can also become affected due to their becoming compressed as a result of pressure from tissue-swelling in and around the eyeballs (orbital areas). With this condition that can be present with TED, a patient may experience pain, inability to see colors and/or partial loss of vision which will affect one or both eyes. Nerve cell damage may occur with optic neuropathy and eventual blindness is possible if treatment for TED is delayed.

The Role of Myxedema in TED

Myxedema is a term meaning tissues in the body are retaining fluid (edema) and a build-up of mucin (mucus) will cause a thickening of the skin in areas of the body, or what is also referred to as "pretibial mucinosis". The condition is often present in autoimmune thyroid disease patients who are experiencing TED. Areas on the face can become swollen for example and will have a puffy appearance. The deep tissues around the eyes can also become swollen as well as tissues behind the eyes. This causes less area in the eye-sockets for movement and to retain the orbital position of the eyes, causing them to be pushed forward and to protrude.

Treatments for TED

The first line of treatment when TED is diagnosed is to correct any thyroid hormone imbalance that might be present if it is not already being done. In cases when thyroid autoimmunity is the cause of hyperthyroidism, patients may need to have their thyroid glands removed. Some medical research studies state that surgical removal of the gland (thyroidectomy) may be a better choice than destruction of the gland by radioactive iodine (ablation) because of the risk the latter mentioned procedure may present to some patients with TED, in worsening the condition.

The following list of treatments may also be administered individually or in combination as determined by a treating physician.

• Prescription eye drops for added lubrication to help prevent dryness and redness.

• Corticosteroid (cortical steroid) and/or topical hydrocortisone to reduce inflammation in the eyes and in tissues surrounding the eyes.

• Radiotherapy or Decompression Surgery (possibly both) to reduce pressure in the eyeballs and to prevent potential damage to them.

• Surgery for lengthening the eyelids that do not fully cover the eyes due to protrusion of them.

• TED patients who are smokers can benefit by quitting due to chemicals in cigarettes that cause inflammation in the eyes and may also be a recommendation by their doctors.

CHAPTER EIGHT

Symptoms and Manifestations of Thyroid Storm

The Hyperthyroid Condition Requiring Emergency Care

Thyroid Storm is a condition in which a thyroid patient experiences sudden, severe hyperthyroidism that requires emergency treatment to prevent injury or death.

This disorder of extremely severe hyperthyroid symptoms is rare but due to its potential to cause bodily injury through damage to organs and possible coma or death, all thyroid patients should have general knowledge about signs and symptoms of Thyroid Storm.

Symptoms

The symptoms of Thyroid Storm will occur suddenly and with extreme force. They are the symptoms of hyperthyroidism but some of the manifestations of the condition are not typical of common overactive thyroid conditions. The general symptoms of severe hyperthyroidism include very rapid heart (tachycardia), extreme nervousness and anxiety, chronic diarrhea, uncontrollable energy, severe hypertension and muscle weakness.

The non-typical symptoms of Thyroid Storm that occur with other severe hyperthyroid symptoms include mental confusion, psychosis (hallucinations and delusions), severe vomiting, unusual behaviors, a sudden high fever, heart arrhythmias that can progress to cardiac arrest and fainting spells. These less common symptoms are likely the ones that would point to something beyond a phase of typical hyperthyroidism. When these signs and symptoms appear, the patient should be taken into emergency medical care immediately, to prevent coma and/or death from occurring.

Is Thyroid Storm Exclusive to Hyperthyroid Patients?

No, the condition can also occur in hypothyroid patients although it is more common in those with hyperthyroidism, especially the autoimmune-caused type called Graves' disease. Patients with hypothyroidism caused by Hashimoto's (autoimmune thyroiditis) have also been known to experience Thyroid Storm and those patients who experience intermittent phases of hyperthyroidism referred to as "Hashitoxicosis" are at higher risk for having a Thyroid Storm.

Causes and Triggers

When Thyroid Storm occurs, the T3 and T4 thyroid hormones elevate to very high levels, causing severe thyrotoxicity (toxic levels). Graves' disease patients and others who are being treated for hyperthyroidism can experience Thyroid Storm if they suffer a heart attack or a severe infection in their bodies. Any traumatic experience can result in this condition of severe hyperthyroidism, including accidents that cause severe physical trauma. Patients treated for hypothyroidism can experience the condition, if they are given excessively high levels of thyroid hormone replacement that causes their T4 and/or T3 levels to elevate far above normal values.

Treatments

The treatments for Thyroid Storm include those that are typical for treating hyperthyroidism but in this case the drugs that are administered must be done at higher doses until symptoms are brought under control. If a hyperthyroid patient has already received treatments to shut down their own thyroid hormone production (thyroid removal) and they are taking thyroid hormone therapy, the replacement hormone must be discontinued while treatment is given.

The treating physician will increase or begin administering levels of anti-thyroid drugs (to reduce thyroid hormone levels) and beta-blocker medications that calm hypertensive and cardiac arrhythmia symptoms. Anti-inflammatory drugs may also be needed to reduce inflammation and fever levels. This may include powerful corticosteroids (steroid anti-inflammatory) and/or over-the-counter drugs that reduce inflammation. Patients are closely monitored until symptoms of Thyroid Storm have diminished and there is no danger of relapse.

CHAPTER NINE

Support for Struggling Thyroid Patients

Two Reasons Why Information and Support Resources are Important

1. Newly diagnosed thyroid patients often express the fact that despite quality treatment for thyroid disease, their doctors do not have the ability due to time-constraints, to fully inform them about their disease/disorder. Most patients feel a great need to understand what is happening to them (self-education) because the unknown aspects of thyroid problems can create fear and frustration in many patients.

2. Thyroid patients experience serious bouts of emotional issues from thyroid disease (anxiety and/or depression) and from the realities of experiencing the onset of a disease that will affect them, for the rest of their lives. A source of emotional support, such as a doctor, is not available to a patient, at any time a need might arise but only for a few minutes, at office visits that are relatively infrequent. Patients can feel very alone with their disease and even those closest to them, may be at a loss for knowing how to support and comfort them.

The facts addressed in these two points alone help to point out the purpose and importance for the availability of information and support resources, that can be shared between thyroid patients. Fellow-patients can often relate better to each other than they can to their own healthy family members.

It is unfortunate when patients are told that they should not look into support resources online because they "might be led astray with wrong information" and that they should somehow rely solely on their doctor, not only for treatment but also for needed, general education about their disease and the often-needed support for coping with it.

Getting these needs met by a treating doctor is simply not possible in most cases, unless a patient's spouse or close relative is a doctor. In the case of a patient who doesn't especially feel the need for information and support, it wouldn't be necessary to begin with but for many patients it can actually mean survival if they are seriously affected by their disease. It is sometimes forgotten that complications from thyroid disease can include things such as Thyroid

Eye Disease, Obstructive Goiters, chronic mood disorders and Thyroid Storm (potentially life threatening).

Most thyroid patients have the common sense to learn from reputable sources when doing an online search about their disease and to the compare information they find with other reliable sources, so that it is confirmed. At many thyroid disease forums and message boards for example, patients share general information that can be confirmed by reputable source-links, plus they can offer support that comes from fellow-patient experience.

To deny patients this type help, for fear of them being led astray by incorrect information etc..., could mean tremendous lost opportunities for patients who have serious struggles coping with their thyroid disease.

CHAPTER TEN

Coping with Thyroid Disease

Methods for Dealing with a Lifetime Health Disorder

Educate Yourself about your Thyroid Disorder

Being newly diagnosed with a thyroid disease or disorder can be concerning and can sometimes create more anxiety in a person when they feel less informed about what is happening to them. Doctors do not always have enough time to thoroughly educate their patients about their diagnosis due to having large numbers of patients to treat as mentioned previously. Some doctors help educate their patients by providing them with informative brochures about their thyroid conditions.

In addition to information your doctor provides, you can also search online for information that will help generally educate you. Reputable and reliable sources are a great way to become better informed about symptoms, treatment and any risks for developing other related problems from your thyroid disorder. Some of the better thyroid information sources include the AACE (American Association of Clinical Endocrinologists), MedLinePlus (National Institutes of Health), WebMD and the ATA (American Thyroid Association).

Join Fellow Patient Thyroid Forums and Support Groups

You can get connected to other thyroid patients by joining forums and groups that offer support to thyroid patients. Many of these forums are volunteer and non-profit. Others do make money from ad space they sell or share but many times this is to help run the forum or group they moderate or administrate and to cover any expenses.

By corresponding with other thyroid patients through these types of resources, you can hear their personal stories and possibly relate-to many of the things they may struggle with in regard to symptoms. You may also hear pointers for getting the best possible treatment for optimal recovery of your health and a better quality of life. There are a number of thyroid forums available, but two of the more reputable are the MedHelp International and HealthBoards thyroid disease forums.

Be Proactive in your Treatment and become a Partner with your Doctor

This simply means you are advocating representing yourself in getting the best possible treatment for your thyroid disease from your doctor. This is better accomplished by first becoming educated about your thyroid disease as mentioned in step one above. A doctor must hear as much as they can from their patient because we are the only person who can let him know how well our treatment is relieving our symptoms.

Doctors are also usually open to suggestions from patients who may feel they need a certain test run to better evaluate how well their treatment is going or in suggesting a change in the dose-level of a medication they are receiving. Of course this type partnering needs to be done in balance so that your doctor doesn't feel that you are not placing trust in him in administering proper treatment. Your goal is simply to help him know how your treatment is going and what you would reasonably like to see accomplished for you over time.

Help to Educate other Thyroid Patients

By referring fellow patients to helpful resources you have received a benefit from and by sharing your personal story you can help to educate them. Sharing the same type of support you have received can serve as a type of therapy in your own continued coping as well. Some thyroid patients, such as me, will begin to compose articles in contributing toward fellow patient education by helping share helpful and general information.

This type of help is sometimes referred to as "Thyroid Patient Advocacy" because the advocate helping fellow patients is also a thyroid patient. Some patients relate better to those who are going through the same or similar experience than they can to their healthy family members or even their own doctors. Doctors can be excellent at treating thyroid diseases, but when it comes to support and coping, fellow patients can sometimes be the best source.

If you are a struggling or a newly diagnosed thyroid patient, consider searching online for helpful information, support and sources that can help you better-cope and regain a better quality of life. It is my hope that this ebook has been a resource that has already contributed toward that goal and I extend my sincere appreciation and best wishes to each reader!

SECTION THREE: **Everything about Thyroid Disease**

CHAPTER ONE

How Many Americans Suffer Thyroid Disorders?

Statistics Reveal Thyroid Disease is Common in the USA

Thyroid diseases and disorders of all types affect millions of Americans and many more people worldwide. The statistics will be addressed in the following subheadings.

According to statistics by the American Association of Clinical Endocrinologists (AACE) and other medical organizations, approximately twenty-seven million Americans are experiencing a thyroid disorder. This includes the estimate that about half of these cases remain undiagnosed.

Thyroid Disease the most common Endocrine Disorder

When compared to the AACE statistics for Americans who experience diabetes, which is approximately sixteen million, the number of people with thyroid disease exceeds that by more than 40%. This makes thyroid disease, the most common endocrine disorder (problem affecting hormone glands) in the USA. Approximately 80% of thyroid disease is experienced by females and women are five times more likely to develop hypothyroidism (an under-active thyroid) than are men.

When all combined, about eight out of ten thyroid disease cases (80%) are hypothyroid conditions with the other two out of ten (20%) being hyperthyroid conditions. As many as two out of ten people who develop diabetes will also experience the onset of a thyroid disorder.

Hereditary and Age-related Risks for Thyroid Disorders

The risk for developing thyroid disease increases when a person is the offspring of at least one parent with thyroid disease. The risk is placed at approximately 50%, meaning about half of all children who have parents with a thyroid disorder, will develop one themselves by the age of 40. The most common age of onset for thyroid disease is between 35 and 40 years. Age-related hypothyroidism can occur at age 60-years and older, with at least 15% of senior-age women and at least 8% of senior-age men developing under-active thyroid glands.

The Risk During and After Pregnancy

Pregnancy also increases the risk for developing hypothyroidism, with approximately 2% of pregnant women experiencing low functioning thyroid glands. This also increases the risk for their newborns to have congenital hypothyroidism (at birth), with statistics placing one-in-five-thousand infants born with under-active thyroids. If "newborn screening" is not done (blood thyroid testing), congenital hypothyroidism can be left undiagnosed and untreated in newborns and can result in slowed development and learning disorders.

Following pregnancy, women are at higher risk for developing postpartum hypothyroidism (one in six) which can develop as much as one-year following giving birth. Up to 25% of these postpartum cases will require lifelong treatment.

Thyroid Autoimmunity, Nodules, Goiters and Cancer

Approximately 10% of Americans test positive for thyroid antibodies. These are the "anti-thyroidperoxidase" and "anti-thyroglobulin" antibodies that are present in both autoimmune hypothyroid and hyperthyroid conditions. Only about 1% of people who test positive for thyroid autoimmunity have full-blown thyroid hormone imbalances, with up to 10% having borderline or subclinically abnormal thyroid hormone levels.

About 40% of confirmed hyperthyroidism cases are caused by Graves' disease (autoimmune hyperthyroidism) affecting approximately 1% of the US population or about 3 million people. In comparison, about 14 million Americans are experiencing Hashimoto's thyroiditis (autoimmune hypothyroidism) and the condition accounts for about 95% of confirmed hypothyroid cases in the US and in other industrialized countries.

Thyroid nodules in general are found in up to half (50%) of the general population. Only 5 to 10 percent of thyroid disease cases involve malignancy (cancer) and only 10% of suspicious thyroid nodules (tumors) are found to be malignant.

Goiters (swollen thyroid glands) are less common in the USA, being experienced by approximately 5% of Americans and many of these do not involve thyroid hormone imbalance. When looked at worldwide, approximately 740 million people are experiencing goiters with approximately 50 million cases being caused by iodine deficiency, a cause that is rare in the USA.

Iodine deficiency is the most common cause of hypothyroidism worldwide, affecting populations that consume inadequate amounts of iodine that is absent from table salt and foods in their diets.

CHAPTER TWO

Major Thyroid Disease Causing Antibodies

Auto-Antibodies in Graves' and Hashimoto's

Thyroid autoimmunity is the most common cause of thyroid disease in industrialized countries, causing overactive and under-active hormone disorders.

Thyroid antibodies attack key proteins in the thyroid gland and in some cases, stimulate production of excessive amounts of hormone. These killer cells that are manufactured by the immune system become confused for reasons yet to be fully understood by medical science and they begin to identify thyroid cells as threats in the body. As they attack these cells, the thyroid gland becomes damaged, resulting in inflammation, enlargement of the gland and thyroid hormone imbalances.

Protein-Enzyme Cell Destroying Antibodies

The antibodies, also called "auto-antibodies", that enter into thyroid protein-enzymes, causing destruction of them, are called the "Anti-thyroidperoxidase" and the "Anti-thyroglobulin". Abbreviations commonly used for these on medical blood lab documents are "TPO ABs" and "TG ABs" or "Anti-TPO" and "Anti-TG".

Once these proteins called thyroidperoxidase and thyroglobulin are destroyed by these antibodies, they are rendered incapable of aiding in the process of converting iodine absorbed by the thyroid gland, into thyroid hormones that regulate the metabolism of all other cells in the body. This is the rate at which the body burns fuels that enter the body, converting them into energy.

As less hormone becomes available the metabolism can be slowed down (hypothyroidism). These proteins are also part of what keeps thyroid tissue healthy and so as the level of them begins to diminish, thyroid tissue will also begin to die within the gland. As this process occurs, the thyroid gland can become inflamed (thyroiditis) and/or enlarged (goiter).

Thyroid Stimulating Antibodies

These antibodies are also called "Thyroid Stimulating Immunoglobulins" (abbreviated TSI). These type auto-antibodies stimulate excessive release of T3-triiodothyronine and T4-thyroxine from the thyroid gland. They do this by binding to receptors in the blood that normally attach to the Thyroid Stimulating Hormone (TSH) which is another hormone that comes from the pituitary brain-gland that regulates hormone release from the thyroid gland.

TSH in-essence is a messenger hormone, telling the thyroid gland how much hormone is needed in the body and keeps the levels in-balance for proper metabolism via ongoing communication. Once the TSI antibodies attach to TSH-receptors, the message from them to the thyroid gland mimics the communication of TSH which stimulates an increase in thyroid hormone levels. They are in-essence tricking the thyroid gland into producing more thyroid hormone when it is not needed, causing a sped up metabolism in the body (hyperthyroidism).

Graves' Disease and Hashimoto's Thyroiditis

All three types of antibodies described in the previous subheadings can be present in both Graves' disease and Hashimoto's thyroiditis. Graves', results in eventual hyperthyroidism in most cases and Hashimoto's results in hypothyroidism. The diseases are differentiated and diagnosed by the balance of auto-antibodies found, by levels of thyroid hormones in the body (imbalances) and by the symptom manifestations caused by the combination of these two factors.

The TPO and TG antibodies are typically found in higher titers (lab measurements) in Hashimoto's patients than in Graves' patients, so both diseases cause thyroid gland destruction but at a much slower rate with Graves' disease. The TSI antibodies that stimulate excessive hormone release from the thyroid gland are found to be high-positive in the vast majority of Graves' patients but are not found to be positive in all Hashimoto's patients and when they are, it is usually in low titers. If a Hashimoto's patient does have significant levels of TSI, it can cause, intermittent phases of hyperthyroidism, called "Hashitoxicosis" which is most often a temporary condition.

These facts about antibodies point to how closely related Graves' and Hashimoto's are and may also explain as to why patients with one disease may transition over to the other in rare cases when a significant change in the balance of auto-antibodies and thyroid hormone levels takes place.

CHAPTER THREE

Major Triggers for Thyroid Autoimmunity

Reasons the Immune System Attacks the Thyroid

Thyroid autoimmunity is a major cause of thyroid disease in industrialized countries. Environmental pollutants and toxins, viral exposure and stress can all be factors.

Thyroid autoimmunity is a term describing the process whereby the immune system creates and sends auto-antibodies to attack proteins in the thyroid gland. These thyroid antibodies cause damage to the gland over time which eventually results in thyroid hormone imbalance. Autoimmune thyroid conditions are also considered to be inflammatory diseases and can also result in goiter, thyroid nodules (small tumors) and other symptoms, in advance of thyroid hormone abnormalities.

Viruses

Some medical research conclusions have cited the Epstein-Barr virus (EBV) as a possible cause of autoimmune thyroid disease. The research studies state that patients with autoimmune thyroiditis tested positive for blood levels of EBV antigens, significantly more often in the thyroid disease group than in the healthy control group. While EBV was the virus studied, there are a number of possible viruses that can trigger autoimmune diseases in susceptible individuals.

Many of these viruses, especially those in the herpes family, are contracted in early life and carried life-long. It may be that the immune system's failure to fully eradicate the body of these viruses causes it to begin attacking organs or tissues in the body that contain the virus, including the thyroid gland. Some patients, who develop sub-acute thyroiditis (temporary) that is often triggered by respiratory viruses, go on to develop permanent autoimmune thyroiditis. It may be that these individuals were predisposed to develop thyroid disease once exposed to any number of possible triggers.

Environmental Toxins

Research studies on possible causes of thyroid autoimmunity have also proposed the possibility of environmental toxins as being a common cause for the immune system attacking the thyroid gland. As the body accumulates these toxins, which the body recognizes as allergens or as strong intolerances, the immune system is triggered in trying to control these things that are in-essence acting as poisons in the body.

Elevated levels of radioactivity (ionizing radiation), such as may be experienced by those who work at nuclear power facilities or at x-ray imaging labs that are over-exposed or not properly protected, can develop autoimmune thyroid diseases. This type of toxin has been well-substantiated as a cause, including studies of children exposed to radiation following the 1986 Chernobyl nuclear power plant accident in Ukraine that caused radioactive fallout. A significant number of children and young adults tested positive for thyroid antibodies in studies conducted 6 to 8 years following the accident.

Other toxins and pollutants that have been studied and that are considered strong possibilities for causing thyroid autoimmunity include toxins found in our water systems, additives and preservatives found in manufactured foods and excessive exposure to fluoride.

Stress

Chronic stress has been studied in relation to many diseases and proposed as a cause for them. This includes inflammatory and autoimmune diseases, types of cancers and immune deficiency illnesses including Chronic Fatigue Syndrome and Fibromyalgia. Many thyroid patients report that they experienced a severe or prolonged period of stress (chronic) just before the onset of their autoimmune thyroid diseases.

This association has been better substantiated in patients studied who have Graves' disease, the autoimmune-caused hyperthyroid condition. While less, studies cite stress as a factor in Hashimoto's thyroiditis patients, it would seem obvious that a triggered autoimmune response can result in either condition because all types of thyroid auto-antibodies can be found in both types of thyroid diseases.

CHAPTER FOUR

Thyroid Autoimmunity and Joint Pain

Rheumatic Symptoms of Thyroid Disease

Muscle and joint aches and stiffness can be chronic in some thyroid patients. These rheumatic symptoms may need special attention if unrelieved with thyroid treatment.

Joint and muscle aches are a common manifestation of thyroid disorders of both the hyperthyroid and hypothyroid types. Medical research on the connection of rheumatic symptoms to thyroid disorders has revealed that it can be a result of "thyroid autoimmunity" rather than thyroid hormone imbalance alone. The studies also make mention of the fact that some patients whose thyroid imbalances are corrected to a euthyroid state, meaning normal thyroid hormone levels, may continue to experience a degree of rheumatic symptoms.

Fibromyalgia often associated with Thyroid Disorders

Patients with fibromyalgia syndrome (FMS) are often found to have a degree of thyroid dysfunction or thyroid autoimmunity (antibodies) and some statistics have shown this connection to be as high as in 75% of cases. A diagnostic, criteria for FMS, are "tender points", which are various points on the body where muscles attach to bones and these are painful when pressed-on with a fingertip.

FMS can be diagnosed when a patient is found to have at least 11 tender points in the body. Hypothyroid patients also report experiencing these tender points when their thyroid hormone levels become low due to a need for a thyroid hormone dose increase, while others continue to experience them even when well-treated. This fact demonstrates the importance in doctors who suspect FMS in patients, ordering thyroid function tests to further evaluate them.

Rheumatic Symptoms when Adjusting to a Thyroid Hormone Dose

There is an adjustment period that occurs when newly treated hypothyroid patients are started on a dose of thyroid replacement hormone. Rheumatic symptoms affecting muscle and joints can flare during this period of adjustment to thyroid hormone coming into the body from an outside source (oral dosing). For most patients the adjustment side-effects resolve in about an eight-week period but for others, their bodies may take longer to adjust to a new dose. This can also be true of a patient already being treated, who is given a dose increase or decrease in follow-up to their monitored treatment. Once the thyroid dose is fully adjusted-to, rheumatic symptoms should improve significantly or resolve completely.

Treatment for Unresolved Rheumatic Symptoms in Thyroid Patients

If joint and muscle aches, stiffness, swelling or redness continues in thyroid patients who are well-treated, their doctor may need to thoroughly evaluate them for the possibility of other rheumatic diseases being present. If thyroid disease is the autoimmune type, a patient is at higher risk for developing other autoimmune diseases, including Rheumatoid Arthritis. If these type conditions and their needed treatments are ruled out, the treatment for thyroid-related rheumatic symptoms would be that used to treat mild forms of arthritis.

Over-the-counter anti-inflammatory medications can help relieve symptoms, as well as mild well-tolerated exercise that, keeps joints and muscles stretched and mobile. Supplementing with Glucosamine and Chondroitin, two natural remedies has been shown to improve rheumatic and arthritic conditions. Getting plenty of rest and sleep can also help keep inflammation levels better controlled. A diet low in refined sugar and rich in foods containing "Beta-cryptoxanthin" and "Zeaxanthin" (carotenoids) can also be beneficial in relieving rheumatic conditions. These would be fruits containing orange and yellow colors and green-leafy vegetables.

CHAPTER FIVE

Chronic Anxiety Associated with Thyroid Disorder

Symptoms of Anxiety Induced by Thyroid Disease

Chronic anxiety symptoms are common in both hypothyroid and hyperthyroid conditions. The cause can be rooted in both hormone imbalance and thyroid autoimmunity.

An overactive thyroid gland or "hyperthyroidism" often causes anxiety symptoms, due to an abnormal increase of metabolism in the body. The thyroid sets the metabolic rate of every cell in the body via hormones produced by the gland. When the levels of hormones increase to abnormally high levels (thyrotoxicity), the metabolism becomes speeded up, causing all organs in the body to operate at overdrive, including the endocrine system (glands that release hormones). This means the body's response to burning energy sources coming into the body, including food and oxygen is over-reactive, so that these are used faster than the body normally needs them (hyper-metabolism and hyperventilation).

The rate at which the pancreas regulates glucose (blood sugar) via release of the hormone insulin is also increased as are hormones from the adrenal gland including adrenaline which sets the rate of blood pressure and heart function (pulse). The combination of all of these functions and mechanisms running abnormally high causes symptoms of increased energy, nervousness and anxiety symptoms. People with hyperthyroidism experience a generalized increase in free-floating anxiety, a feeling of being on edge and periods of suddenly escalated anxiety called panic attacks.

Hashitoxicosis from Hashimoto's thyroiditis

Most cases of hypothyroidism in industrialized countries are caused by an autoimmune condition called "Hashimoto's thyroiditis". The under-functioning of the thyroid gland in cases of Hashimoto's, is a result of auto-antibodies that are created and released by the immune system, to attack proteins found in the thyroid gland, causing cell death and eventual damage to the gland. Once enough damage has occurred, the thyroid gland's ability to produce sufficient amounts of hormones is diminished.

"Hashitoxicosis" is an intermittent period of hyperthyroidism experienced by some patients with Hashimoto's. As the hyperthyroid phases occur, sudden and severe anxiety symptoms may manifest, as well as other symptoms of hyperthyroidism. Types of temporary thyroiditis (sub-acute), that are non-autoimmune related that can occur in pregnant women and in people with respiratory viruses can also cause short term hyperthyroidism.

Medical research studies state that Hashitoxicosis does not have to occur for anxiety symptoms to be caused by Hashimoto's, the permanent type thyroiditis but have concluded that anxiety may be associated with the "thyroid autoimmunity" itself.

Hot Thyroid Nodules and Toxic Diffuse Goiters

Tumors may develop in the thyroid gland, called "nodules" and these can be the type that, become "hot", meaning they release thyroid hormone as if they have become part of the gland. When these type nodules become active enough to cause hyperthyroidism, anxiety symptoms may be a part of the symptom-complex that results, as with hyperthyroidism of other causes.

In some patients, the thyroid gland becomes enlarged with or without containing thyroid nodules. This is referred to as a goiter but the gland may also become toxic (overactive) as a result of the goiter, which is referred to as a "toxic diffuse goiter". Most people with autoimmune-caused hyperthyroidism or "Graves' disease" have toxic diffuse goiters. If there is a combination of goiter and nodules, it may be referred to as a multi-nodular - toxic diffuse goiter.

Treatment for Anxiety caused by Thyroid Disorders

For most cases of anxiety symptoms related to thyroid disorders, treating the disorder itself will bring relief of symptoms or even complete resolution of them. In cases of autoimmune-related hypothyroidism, replacing the low hormone levels, will correct the metabolism and help to reduce or control the thyroid antibody levels. In cases of hyperthyroidism, regardless of cause, reducing thyroid hormone levels using "anti-thyroid" and/or "beta-blocker" medications will reduce or resolve symptoms in some cases.

In more severe cases of hyperthyroidism, that cannot be controlled with these type drugs partial or full thyroid removal (thyroidectomy surgery) may be necessary or destruction of the gland by radioactive iodine (ablation). Removal of part or all of the thyroid gland may also be required in cases of hot nodules and toxic diffuse goiters.

If these treatments still do not relieve anxiety symptoms, anti-anxiety medications or SSRI antidepressants may be prescribed. Therapies to help patients cope with anxiety may also be recommended, such as "Cognitive Behavioral Therapy", which has been found to be a very effective treatment for anxiety conditions.

CHAPTER SIX

Understanding the T3 and T4 Thyroid Hormones

Facts about Thyroxine and Triiodothyronine

The two major thyroid hormones are called "thyroxine" (T4) and "triiodothyronine" (T3). Their purpose is to regulate the rate of metabolism in every cell of the body.

The thyroid gland consists largely of iodine and from it, produces the T4 and T3 thyroid hormones. This process is accomplished in the liver and kidneys and within the thyroid hormone cells themselves with the aid of iodide peroxidase enzymes (thyroidperoxidase) and thyroglobulin, which are also referred to as thyroid proteins.

Thyroxine-T4 Converts into T3

Thyroxine, known as the T4, is the one most abundant in the body representing approximately 80% of thyroid hormones but is also a precursor to T3. While medical research shows that T4 does have a purpose at the tissue-level, in regulating bodily metabolism, its other major function as a "prohormone" is to convert into the T3 hormone (triiodothyronine).

There are four iodine molecules in T4 but it loses one of the atoms (single element) of iodine from these molecules (combined elements), which is removed from its outer ring once converted into T3 which will then have three iodine molecules. The T3 it converts into is at least four times more powerful in spite of having one-less iodine molecule and is more active in regulating bodily metabolism. When looked at it from this point of view, T4 is less active, with the purpose of being on stand-by as a reserve hormone, to be converted into the active T3 as needed in the body.

Excess Triiodothyronine-T3 is converted into Reverse T3

T3 represents approximately 20% of thyroid hormones found in the body. When the body has enough T3 available, any excess T4 remaining in reserve, will be rendered inactive by the conversion of it into "Reverse T3" (RT3). This process is ongoing due to the fact that the thyroid gland continues to absorb iodine from things consumed in the diet, from which to continue producing hormones. In the case of T4 being converted into RT3, one iodine atom is removed from the inner ring of the iodine molecules. This process which also occurs mainly in the liver and kidneys is a safe-guard against over-stimulation of bodily metabolism from an excess of T3 hormone or "hyperthyroidism".

Low T3 Syndrome

In some cases a disease process in the body, a medication being taken or chronic stress, can cause excessive conversion of T4 into RT3 and this will cause T3 levels to drop too low, causing hypothyroidism. While this cause of low T3 is rare, it does occur and is referred to by several names, including "Low T3 Syndrome", "Euthyroid Sick Syndrome", "Reverse T3 Syndrome" and "Wilson's Temperature Syndrome". In most cases of excessive RT3 conversion, the hypothyroidism is temporary and can be corrected by supplementing short-term with T3 hormone and correcting the problem in the body causing the condition.

Impaired Conversion of T4 into T3

Usually when a person becomes hypothyroid, the T4 itself becomes low but because it is the forerunner to the manufacture of T3, this in turn causes both levels to become low over time. In some cases however, adequate T4 will be produced by the thyroid gland but then fails to be converted into an adequate amount of T3. The term often used for this condition is "impaired conversion" and will cause hypothyroidism due to a lack of the more metabolically active T3 hormone.

As mentioned in the previous subheading, the resulting condition is referred to as "Low T3 Syndrome" but in this case it is due to failure of conversion of T4 into T3. The condition cannot be detected by testing the TSH level alone (pituitary hormone that reflects thyroid levels) but tests of the T4 and T3 must be ordered to detect the problem. The impairment can be due to a number of factors but in some cases may be due to kidney and/or liver disease, the organs in which the conversion process takes place.

In addition to organ problems, an autoimmune disease process affecting thyroid function may result in a lack of iodide peroxidase enzymes and/or thyroglobulin. The antibodies that attack these enzymes/proteins are called the anti-thyroidperoxidase (Anti-TPO) and the anti-thyroglobulin (anti-TG).

CHAPTER SEVEN

Understanding the TSH Hormone

The Function of Thyroid Stimulating Hormone

The pituitary-gland hormone called "Thyroid Stimulating Hormone" (TSH) is highly sensitive in detecting thyroid hormone imbalances earlier than any other blood test.

Thyroid Stimulating Hormone (TSH) is the most commonly used blood lab-tested hormone level in evaluating thyroid function. It is highly sensitive and able to detect thyroid hormone imbalances earlier than any other blood test. There are other interesting facts about this important endocrine hormone that will be addressed in the following subheadings.

TSH is not a Thyroid Hormone

TSH actually comes from one of the master brain-glands called the "pituitary gland". It is the hormone that stimulates thyroid hormone production. The hormones released from the thyroid gland (T4 and T3) once responding to stimulation by TSH are the ones the regulate bodily metabolism. As the need for thyroid hormone fluctuates during a 24 hour period, the TSH level can change by as much as 2-points but will stay within normal values if there is not a problem within the thyroid gland.

TSH Rises when the Thyroid Gland is Under-Functioning

If the pituitary gland senses that there is not enough thyroid hormone being released (hypothyroidism) due to the gland struggling or being hindered by a disease process, it will send an excess of TSH to further stimulate thyroid hormone production. This is the point at which lab values of blood-tested TSH levels will usually be flagged high and will continue to rise as the hypothyroidism worsens. The hormone level will be sensitive enough, so that even mild, sub-clinical cases of hypothyroidism will be detected early into the development of them.

Normal values range between blood testing labs but an approximate average of the low-normal range for TSH is between 0.3 and 0.5 and the high-normal range averages between 3.0 and 5.0.

TSH Falls with an Over-Functioning Thyroid Gland

The opposite effect will occur when the thyroid gland is producing too much thyroid hormone (hyperthyroidism). The pituitary gland will back-off and send less of the stimulating hormone when the thyroid is overactive. This is the pituitary gland's attempt to prevent worsening of the hyperthyroidism and if overproduction of thyroid hormones is severe, TSH may actually become undetectable when blood testing the level. Both a low-normal TSH and a high-normal TSH or borderline levels on either end of the normal values merits follow-up blood retesting because sub-normal levels can be an indication of a developing thyroid hormone disorder.

TSH does not Detect Thyroid Disease

This amazing endocrine hormone, with its great sensitivity, actually does not diagnose the "cause" of an over-functioning or an under-functioning thyroid gland. Blood levels of TSH are valuable in detecting thyroid hormone imbalances but further testing is required to find the cause of a thyroid hormone imbalance. A disease process in the thyroid gland will most often be the cause of an abnormal TSH reading.

There are however, other possible causes of TSH imbalance, including a tumor or disease process occurring within the pituitary gland itself and thyroid hormone imbalances due to a medication a person is taking or another disease process in the body not directly related to the thyroid gland. These types of causes affecting thyroid hormone levels are very rare compared to thyroid diseases.

Follow up blood testing of other thyroid-related levels may help to determine the cause of an abnormal TSH level and thyroid hormone imbalances. This includes testing for "thyroid antibodies" that can detect autoimmunity in the gland (immune system response) and testing the actual T3 and T4 thyroid hormone levels. Thyroid disease cases involving goiters or thyroid nodules may also require imaging tests or tissue biopsies.

CHAPTER EIGHT

Thyroid Disease Problem-Symptoms

Problems That Can Linger Despite Proper Treatment

Treatments for thyroid disorders and diseases can be very effective. There are however particular symptoms that can continue to cause problems in some patients.

The symptoms of both hypothyroidism and hyperthyroidism are varied and sometimes very serious. Some symptoms are common with both types of disorders or what might be called "crossover symptoms".

Common Symptoms of Thyroid Hormone Imbalances

The typical symptoms of both hypothyroidism and hyperthyroidism are usually significantly improved with treatments for each. "Problem-symptoms" would be those that are not as typical and that often require additional attention to see significant resolution for them. Following are lists of common symptoms for both hypothyroid and hyperthyroid disorders.

Hyperthyroidism – is a condition involving elevated thyroid hormone levels that increases metabolism to an abnormally sped-up level. Hyperthyroid symptoms include increased energy, nervousness, rapid weight loss, sweating, tremor (trembling), rapid heart rate and breathing, difficulty sleeping, heat intolerance, goiter and increased bowel movements and urination.

Hypothyroidism – is the opposite condition in which thyroid hormone levels drop below normal, causing slowed bodily metabolism. The symptoms of becoming hypothyroid include lack of energy and fatigue, depression, weight gain, dry skin, cold extremities, an increased need to sleep, goiter, difficulty concentrating, feeling slowed down and constipation.

Low Libido

Libido is a term meaning sex-drive and thyroid patients often experience a drop in sexual desire, which can be very concerning when they feel they are not as responsive to the needs of their partners. For male patients this can be more of a problem due to the fact that they may experience erectile dysfunction which causes inability to complete intimacy at the fullest level.

In addition to being reassured by a treating doctor that a patient's thyroid hormone levels are at proper range, there are prescription medications for erectile dysfunction including Viagra, Levitra and Cialis. Natural treatments that can help increase libido in both men and women include Vitamins E and C, flaxseed, arginine (amino acid), the mineral-zinc, bioflavonoids and the herbal supplements - ginkgo biloba and ginseng.

Hair Loss

This problem-symptom is not exclusive to men; in fact thyroid disease is a major cause of hair loss in women. Thyroid hormone imbalances of either hypothyroidism or hyperthyroidism can cause hair to fall out or in some cases to become brittle and break-off. Patients taking thyroid hormone replacement can experience hair loss when first beginning their treatment dose.

As the body better adjusts to the hormone, the hair loss will usually improve or completely resolve. Switching brands after being adjusted to a current one can also cause a phase of hair loss and it seems to be slightly more common in patients taking synthetic brands of thyroid hormone rather than natural brands.

Medications used to treat hair loss include Finasteride and Proscar-Propecia for men and Minoxidil and Aldactone for women. In some cases pattern baldness in both men and women can be caused by adrenal and/or sex hormone imbalances, in which case, a treating doctor would administer additional hormone replacement therapy in addition to treating the thyroid disorder.

Brain Fog

This symptom, often not completely resolved with treatment for thyroid disorder, is in the area of one's ability to concentrate and focus on things requiring mental abilities. Patients report that their concentration lacks the sharpness and clarity they had before the onset of their thyroid disease. Some even report episodes of difficulty in word-retrieval, meaning they find it difficult to complete sentences with the appropriate words or to remember the names of people they are well-acquainted with.

When well-treated thyroid hormone imbalance does not improve brain-fog symptoms, there are lifestyle changes and supplements that can help in this area. Getting proper sleep and rest is very important, as well as improving diet practices by eating healthy foods and eliminating stimulants such as caffeine, alcohol and refined sugar. While these substances can help with energy and concentration short-term, they can also cause energy crashes or what might be referred to as stimulant-hangovers.

Supplements that can increase mental clarity and concentration include CoQ10, selenium, B-vitamins (including folic acid), Vitamin C and E and Omega 3 fatty acids. Herbal supplements that may help in this area include ginkgo biloba and Asian ginseng but any supplements should be approved by a treating physician.

CHAPTER NINE

Skin Problems Associated with Thyroid Disease

Autoimmunity and Hormone Imbalances Affecting the Epidermis

Thyroid diseases and thyroid hormone imbalances can cause changes and/or diseases affecting the epidermis (skin) but treatments are available.
Patients experiencing diseases of the thyroid that involves auto-antibodies directed at the gland and those who experience hyperthyroidism (overactive gland) and hypothyroidism (under-active gland) can potentially develop disorders affecting the skin. There are, however,

treatments that can reduce epidermal symptoms and in many cases, completely resolve them.

Hypothyroidism – Dry Skin

When a person develops hypothyroidism, meaning an under-functioning thyroid gland, there is not an adequate amount of thyroid hormone to sufficiently operate the organ and gland systems of the body. Everything in the body begins to slow down, including the sweat glands (sudoriferous) and oil glands (sebacious) that moisturize and lubricate the outside layers of the skin. This causes dryness of the skin, resulting in cracking and flaking and the need to use moisturizing lotions more often than they are normally needed.

Hyperthyroidism – Oily Skin

The opposite is true when hyperthyroidism develops. Over-production of thyroid hormone causes all bodily systems to begin operating at overdrive due to their being sped-up by an overactive thyroid gland. This results in the sweat glands and oil secreting glands under the skin, producing more of these moisturizing agents than are needed. The skin will become clammy and oily in some cases and blemishes may begin to develop. Some hyperthyroid patients may break out with cases of acne, meaning the blemishes are frequent and widespread on the face or other areas of the body.

Myxedema

Both hypothyroid and hyperthyroid patients can potentially develop "edema of the skin" (non-pitting swelling), a term referring to the increased deposit of components found normally in the deep tissues of the skin. These deposited skin components include:

• glycosaminoglycan

• hyaluronic acid

• mucopolysaccharides

These components are increased secondary to "lymphocytic infiltrate," meaning white blood cells are responding to inflammation in the body, causing the increased skin deposits. The white blood cells involved in this response include:

• neutrophils

• lymphocytes

• monocytes

This inflammatory response can be due to thyroid hormone imbalance and/or "thyroid autoimmunity," which is the attack by auto-antibody cells (thyroid antibodies) sent from the immune system, that mistakenly attacks the thyroid gland. Thyroid related edema is referred to as "myxedema" and in hypothyroid patients can affect any area of the body but will often first be noticeable in the face. Hyperthyroid patients can experience myxedema in any area of their bodies as well but they will often experience it in their lower extremities, below the knees (feet and ankles), called "pretibial edema/myxedema" or "thyroid dermopathy."

Thyroid Autoimmunity

Medical research studies have found that "chronic uticaria," meaning frequent and/or severe flares of hives (prominent rash) can directly result from auto-antibodies that attack the thyroid gland. In this case, the hives may not fully respond to correction of thyroid hormone imbalances that may also be present.

Autoimmune thyroid diseases patients are also at higher risk for developing other autoimmune conditions/diseases of the skin which may include the following:

• Sjögren's Syndrome (chronic dryness)

• vitiligo (patches of loss in pigment)

• eczema (scaly, itchy, crusting or blistering)

• dermatitis herpetiformis (bumpy, blistery rash)

• psoriasis (redness and irritation)

Treatments

In many cases, skin conditions caused by thyroid diseases resolve once the associated thyroid hormone imbalance is corrected. Some cases may require additional treatments of other underlying autoimmune diseases or may require additional prescribed medications. These may include:

• topical hydrocortisone creams

• moisturizing lotions

• antihistamine drugs

A treating thyroid doctor may refer their patients with severe skin problems and those whose skin problems that do not respond well to thyroid treatments, to a dermatologist (skin specialist) for further treatment.

Symptoms affecting the skin often respond well when the associated thyroid disorder is well-treated. When these conditions do not respond well, however, there are additional treatments that can relieve symptoms and in some cases resolve the associated skin disorders. Anyone experiencing symptoms involving their epidermis should see their doctor for further evaluation because it may also reveal other underlying diseases or disorders in the body.

CHAPTER TEN

Mononucleosis and Hashimoto's Thyroiditis

The Epstein-Barr Virus and Thyroid Autoimmunity

Many medical research articles cite the Epstein-Barr Virus as being highly associated with autoimmune diseases, one of these being Hashimoto's thyroiditis.

Medical researchers continue to study autoimmune diseases, in attempt to find definitive causes for them. One virus that continues to be found in higher titers (blood measurements) among autoimmune disease patients, than in the healthy population, is the Epstein-Barr Virus (EBV). One specific medical study concludes that the association of EBV has been found in patients with autoimmune thyroiditis as well.

EBV More Serious Than Once Believed

Medical research has revealed in recent years, that EBV is associated strongly with autoimmune diseases of all types; in fact during the years 2006 through 2008, several medical groups issued press releases including Multiple Sclerosis among the diseases that can be caused or triggered by EBV. Approximately 80% of the general population is infected with EBV.

Even when immunity against EBV initially develops in a person's body, the dormant virus can later go on to cause the onset of chronic, autoimmune or inflammatory diseases in susceptible individuals. The virus is also linked to causing certain types of cancer.

Some People Who Contract EBV Experience Mononucleosis

The initial illness of Mononucleosis (mono) that can result from EBV infection is usually not serious or life-threatening but the viral symptoms of fatigue, body aches and swollen lymph nodes in the neck will require bed rest, increased fluid intake and over-the-counter anti-inflammatory drugs to moderate fever. This illness, also referred to as "the kissing disease" usually resolves within six weeks of contracting it. Many people, who contract the virus and carry it in their bodies lifelong, do not experience the symptoms of mono.

Studies State That EBV Can Reactivate and Replicate

Other medical studies and sources including mentions in articles published by the U.S. National Institutes of Health (PubMed), state that EBV can reactivate and replicate (increase in number) in immunocompromised individuals or what is also referred to as immunodeficiency. Some studies have associated viral reactivation of EBV and other lifetime viruses as being factors in causing Chronic Fatigue Syndrome (also called Myalgic Encephalopathy/ME) which is sometimes referred to as a "post viral illness".

It may also eventually be proven that many thyroid autoimmunity cases are also caused by the EBV virus specifically. It is possible that the immune system's ongoing battle to prevent reactivation and replication of the virus in immuno-compromised individuals results in the eventual turning of the immune system against tissues in the body that contain the virus later in life. Auto-antibodies will be created in these cases, to attack natural parts of the body that are recognized as threats. The continued findings in this area of research will be interesting to follow and may also hold answers to treatments for conditions of autoimmunity in the future.

CHAPTER ELEVEN

Thyroid Disorders Related to Pregnancy

Conditions Affecting the Mother or Baby

Pregnant women are at increased risk for developing thyroiditis and both mother and child can potentially experience thyroid hormone imbalances.

Thyroid inflammation (thyroiditis) can occur in the mother during pregnancy or after giving birth (postpartum). Most cases are temporary and cause a short-term phase of hyperthyroidism – an overactive thyroid gland. Hypothyroidism – an under active thyroid gland – can also develop during pregnancy as much as one year postpartum.

Thyroiditis

The types of thyroiditis that can affect pregnant women include the following:

• silent thyroiditis

• postpartum thyroiditis

• Hashimoto's thyroiditis

• sub-acute/viral thyroiditis

The term "silent" as related to thyroiditis means it is the type that does not cause pain or significant swelling in the thyroid gland, as can the painful type called "sub-acute" that is often related to viral and respiratory infections. Sub-acute or "viral thyroiditis" can, however, also occur during pregnancy if the mother contracts a viral illness. The term "postpartum" simply means the thyroiditis occurs following pregnancy but if it is not painful, and the term "silent" still applies as well.

Pregnancy places extra physical demands on the mother because her body is nourishing the development of a fetus and this requires more activity by the endocrine glands in the body. These are the glands that supply needed hormones, including the thyroid ones that regulate metabolism. The increased demand for more thyroid hormone can result in mild to moderate inflammation in the thyroid gland.

As a result of thyroiditis, the immune system will send cells called "anti-inflammatory cytokines" to moderate the inflammation. Hormones such as "cortisol" (cortical) from the adrenal glands will also increase in the body to help reduce inflammation. This process can take several weeks before the thyroiditis resolves. The thyroid gland itself also attempts to override the inflammation and will become overactive (hyperthyroid) for a couple of weeks following the onset of thyroiditis.

When pregnancy triggers thyroiditis, this can also lead to thyroid autoimmunity or permanent autoimmune thyroiditis (Hashimoto's disease). Temporary types of thyroiditis will usually not cause the mother to test positive for thyroid antibodies or if they are present, they will be found in high-normal or low-positive titers.

Hypothyroidism

Three basic categories of hypothyroidism that can be related to pregnancy are as follows:

• temporary hypothyroidism

• permanent hypothyroidism (usually autoimmune)

• congenital hypothyroidism (neonatal)

For many pregnant mothers, hypothyroidism is a temporary condition but for others it becomes permanent. Factors that affect the type of hypothyroidism that develops include genetic tendency toward thyroid disease, meaning it is passed down through one or both parents and the presence of other endocrine disorders such as diabetes, which can also increase the risk for permanent hypothyroidism.

When a baby is born with hypothyroidism, it is referred to as "congenital hypothyroidism" and in most cases, is a temporary condition. This, points to the importance in blood testing or what is also called "newborn screenings." Treatment for hypothyroidism must be administered in newborns to prevent immature development that can affect them mentally and/or physically.

Risks

Pregnant mothers with thyroid autoimmunity can experiencing high levels of auto-antibodies from the immune system that cause inflammation and damage to the gland. This places them at increased risk for experiencing a miscarriage or having a baby born with birth defects.

If thyroid autoimmunity is discovered prior to pregnancy, mothers wishing to conceive will first be given treatment to reduce the antibody levels and to treat any thyroid hormone imbalance. This will usually require several months of follow-up blood retesting before patients are ready to safely conceive as determined by their doctor.

Treatments

Thyroiditis usually resolves on its own without the need for prescription drugs to control inflammation. Over-the-counter anti-inflammatory drugs (excluding aspirin during pregnancy) are usually all that are necessary, along with sufficient fluid intake and bed rest. If thyroiditis is severe and difficult to resolve, a treating doctor might prescribe an anti-inflammatory steroid called a "corticosteroid," but this treatment would likely be restricted to postpartum cases.

Hypothyroidism in either the mother or baby is treated by replacing the low thyroid hormone by oral or intravenous dosing. Temporary hypothyroidism will resolve after several weeks of a patient receiving a dose of replacement thyroid hormone, while the permanent type will require this as a lifelong treatment.

CHAPTER TWELVE

Mood Disorders in Sub clinical Thyroid Disorder

Emotional Manifestations with Mild Hormone Imbalances

Hypothyroidism is well known for causing depression and hyperthyroidism is well known for causing anxiety symptoms. For some patients these symptoms manifest early.

Both anxiety and depression can manifest as part of the symptom complex in overt (full-blown) hypothyroid and hyperthyroid disorders but some medical studies conclude that emotional symptoms can occur in subclinical cases as well.

Blood Testing Patients with Emotional Disorders

Medical sources on statistics for emotional disorders vary but some place the incidence for depression in the general population at about 20%. Other statistics that separate the numbers by gender state that up to 1 in 4 women (25%) and up to 1 in 6 men (16.6%) will experience a serious bout of depression at some point in their lives. The statistics for anxiety are also very high, with an estimated 18% of the general population experiencing it to a degree serious enough to be called "anxiety disorder", at some point during their adult lives.

Other medical sources state that a significant percentage of emotional disorder cases have underlying medical causes contributing to them or causing them. Health disorders that can cause anxiety and depression symptoms include endocrines ones, such as diabetes, adrenal gland conditions, thyroid disorders, Mitral Valve Prolapse (heart murmur), autoimmune diseases and sex hormone imbalances. With such a variety of potential medical causes being a possibility in emotional symptoms cases, diagnostic blood testing should be a priority to determine if a medical cause exists or if a condition is an emotional-only disorder.

Study Cites Subclincal Thyroid Disorders as a Cause of Anxiety

In a medical research study published on the PubMed website, titled "Assessment of anxiety in subclinical thyroid disorders." the study concludes that anxiety symptoms are significantly increased in patients with subclinical thyroid dysfunction, whether it is of the hyperthyroid or hypothyroid type.

It may be possible that subclinical thyroid hormone imbalance is similar in respect to pre-diabetes and diabetic conditions that can cause hypoglycemia. People, who experience episodes of low glucose (blood sugar), will experience a bodily reaction of increased adrenaline, causing anxiety and nervousness. This is the body's way of compensating one hormone for another that is low or possibly the body's way of trying to encourage more hormone production in the body. It may be that increased adrenaline also occurs to compensate for thyroid hormones that are beginning to head toward low levels (subclinical).

Additional Medical Treatment or Therapies May Still Be Needed

Correcting abnormal thyroid hormone levels can alleviate emotional symptoms in most cases of treatable thyroid dysfunction or significantly reduce them. Subclinical thyroid disorders however, may not be treatable until the hormone imbalance is serious enough to require correction. Hypothyroidism for example that is treated too soon can cause thyrotoxicity by placing more, hormone in the body before it is needed.

Until thyroid treatments can be administered, subclinical thyroid cases may need other drug or psychiatric therapies to control anxiety and/or depression symptoms. These type cases also require repeat blood testing follow ups, to monitor the progression of subclinical thyroid disorders.

CHAPTER THIRTEEN

Disease Acceptance in Thyroid Patients

A Cognitive Behavioral Therapy Coping Method

Thyroid diseases can cause an array of diverse and life-changing symptoms. One aspect of coping for patients is learning to find acceptance for their disease.

Some people who experience the onset of hypothyroid or hyperthyroid disorders find difficulty coping with a health disorder that in most cases requires lifelong treatment. A degree of change in one's ability to carry on with the same level of activities can diminish, causing a thyroid patient to feel disabled to some degree. These type changes can affect a patient emotionally, possibly requiring therapy to help them cope.

Administered Therapies and Self-Therapy

One aspect of emotional therapy that can help patients cope with thyroid disease is one in the "Cognitive Behavioral Therapy" (CBT) category in which patients learn to react differently to changes thyroid symptoms may cause in their lives. Rather than reacting negatively a patient can learn instead, to react with acceptance for something they have no power to change.

Thyroid disease treatments can help tremendously with relief of hormone-imbalance related symptoms but in most cases do not take away certain disease aspects and for some patients a need for coping therapies may arise. Therapy can be administered by mental health professionals in serious cases of emotional coping needs or as self-therapy in patients who have mild to moderate coping needs.

Changes That May Require Emotional Coping

While the general symptoms of thyroid disorders are not always significantly life-changing, others are more severe and can have an emotional impact on patients in a number of ways. Women for example who develop thyroid autoimmunity, are sometimes required to delay pregnancies if they have highly elevated auto-antibody levels and some experience miscarriages due to this problem with autoimmunity.

Other thyroid patients develop Thyroid Eye Disease, in which their eyes bulge and protrude and they can remain in this condition for several years. Others experience significant hair loss or emotional symptoms that can be difficult to resolve and all of these scenarios can be difficult for affected patients to cope with in some cases.

Struggle Increases Stress

The "acceptance" aspect of learning to cope with thyroid disease is similar in-principle to CBT anxiety disorder therapies that teach anxiety sufferers not to struggle with anxiety but to simply learn to flow with it and allow it to take place. In the case of anxiety, continually struggling against symptoms simply fuels them because the "fight or flight" anxiety mechanism thrives on struggle, which serves to repeatedly reactivate them.

The same can be said of patients who struggle against a disease they have no control over, rather than learning to accept it as having become a part of their lives. This type acceptance in the case of a thyroid patient does not mean that he welcomes the disease or approves of it but simply means he accepts the fact that it has entered his life and will remain there unless cured or healed by divine intervention. By strongly resisting a disease with ongoing mental and physical struggle, a patient can actually increase symptoms of stress, anxiety and fatigue.

Giving One's Self Permission to Feel Unwell

A thyroid patient must give himself permission to feel sick if symptoms flare and permission to take extra time to rest and relax. This might also require upfront honesty with friends and relatives who ask for his attendance at events he may not feel able to attend. Simply being honest and saying that the timing is not good for him can help relieve the stress of expectations.

In most cases people are understanding when you explain your reasons to them while others may not be. Regardless, health and wellbeing must always come before pleasing others and a thyroid patient cannot afford to add unnecessary stressors to his life. This same advice can be applied to patients suffering illnesses such as Chronic Fatigue Syndrome and Fibromyalgia.

Medical studies have shown that chronic stress can directly affect thyroid disease severity. In addition to the described CBT coping methods, there are other psychiatric therapies that can help emotionally struggling thyroid patients, as well as medications that can be prescribed by their doctors.

CHAPTER FOURTEEN

Natural Thyroid Treatments and Supplements

Which Ones are Safe to Take?

Many non-prescription products are offered claiming to improve thyroid function. Some are also advertised as treatments for hypothyroidism.

Non-prescription thyroid supplements can contain ingredients such as iodine, l-tyrosine, calcium, phosphate, potassium, olive leaf extract, selenium, guggul extract, processed kelp/seaweed, bioperine, dipotassium phosphate and a number of other varied ingredients.

Some brands are manufactured with processed, porcine (pig) or bovine (cow) thyroid glands added as an ingredient but with the hormones extracted, so that the supplement is hormone-free (to avoid FDA restrictions in applicable countries). Others that contain no thyroid hormone will have names that imply they contain them, when in reality they are also hormone-free.

Deceptive Supplement Marketing Ploys

Many of these supplements contain ingredients that have some benefit in the human body but they have limited affect on thyroid function and the purpose behind the manufacture of them is strictly to gain sales. This is not to say that the vitamins, minerals and healthy ingredients, including herbals don't have a positive effect to a degree in people taking them but the claim that they will improve thyroid function specifically is often exaggerated or completely false. There are other factors that determine how well healthy supplements and nutrients work in the body, including proper diet, exercise and adequate sleep and rest.

Dangerous Stimulants or Ingredients

The common claim by thyroid booster manufacturers is that these supplements increase metabolism in the body via improved thyroid function, which will help the user to lose weight safely. When thyroid boosters contain stimulants however, the user of such a product may feel the energizing effects from the supplement but it s not coming from an increase in thyroid function but is in-essence a stimulant-high that does not result in benefit toward better health or safe weight-loss. In some cases the supplement may instead result in negative effects on health.

Supplements that contain high levels of caffeine or that contain any level of ephedrine or pseudo-amphetamines should be strictly avoided. This is especially true of people who are experiencing hyperthyroidism because these stimulants can worsen the symptoms of an overactive thyroid gland, including increased hypertension and heart arrhythmias.

A similar warning can be applied to supplements containing iodine as well. Some of them add a very high content of iodine as an ingredient that far surpasses the RDA (recommended daily allowance) and medical studies have shown this to be a potential contributing factor toward development of autoimmune thyroid disease in susceptible individuals.

No Substitute for Thyroid Hormone Replacement

Individuals who have hypothyroidism (under-active thyroid) or who have had their thyroid glands removed will afterward require thyroid hormone replacement therapy. A thyroid boosting supplement cannot substitute prescribed thyroid hormone even if it contains iodine as an ingredient because proper levels of thyroid proteins must be present in the body for iodine to be converted into thyroid hormone. This is something that is deficient or missing in people with diseased thyroid glands.

In the case of natural thyroid hormone, some of which can be purchased without a prescription, a qualified doctor will not be prescribing a determined dose by blood test evaluation or monitoring the treatment to adjust the hormones to proper level. This endangers a patient of taking too high a level, causing thyrotoxicity (toxic amount causing hyperthyroidism) or in under-treatment which will allow hypothyroidism to progress and worsen. In short, there is no substitute for thyroid hormone replacement, in patients with hypothyroidism, monitored by a licensed physician administering the treatment.

CHAPTER FIFTEEN

Organizing a Thyroid Disease Support Group

Fellow Patients Sharing Helpful Advice Online or In-Person

Thyroid patients often relate better to fellow-patients who are going through similar struggles to find effective treatments, symptom relieve and best quality-of-life.

Fellow-patient thyroid disease support groups can offer the opportunity for patients to meet and share advice and personal experiences. The benefits of regular meetings in-person or online can also provide opportunity for helpful, reliable resources to be shared among patients who can refer one another to informative books and helpful online information they have found. Meetings can also open discussions on important thyroid topics members may wish to participate in to help them gain general knowledge about their disease and its treatment.

Publicly Announcing a New Support Group

One effective way to inform the public in one's own area about the formation of a new thyroid disease support group is to submit an announcement covering the event in a local newspaper. Local media is often helpful with offering free coverage for something that will be helpful to their community. Written coverage for the support group might be submitted as a letter to the editor, for inclusion in that section or as a news story or press release that contains information in regard to the importance for thyroid patients in the area for such a resource to become available.

The announcement submitter might also consider relating a brief personal story within the submission to the newspaper that demonstrates the need patients have in connecting to other patients and to sources of shared information that can help them cope with their disease emotionally. If a newspaper is reluctant to allow free coverage of the event, a paid advertisement might be a consideration. Local radio stations may also agree to inform the public at no charge by airing announcements for the support group. Typing up flyers on a computer and printing them for distribution to bulletin boards and for handing out can also help get the word out.

Support Group Newsletter

The support group director or those appointed to plan meetings may also consider publishing a monthly or bi-monthly newsletter to inform members about times set for meetings and what information will be covered in them. The newsletter publisher might also offer opportunity for members to submit personal stories and/or helpful information from reliable, reputable sources, for consideration of being added into the newsletter. It can also be offered to the local public in-general whether they decide to become eventual members or not. Personal stories, book reviews and covering discussions taking place in meetings can help gain more interest for the support group. A newsletter can be offered through email and/or in print.

Inviting Guest Speakers

Special guests can be invited to make presentations or to give lectures on thyroid disease subjects for the support group. Area doctors that treat thyroid diseases might be interested in making guest appearances to relate helpful information to thyroid patient members. Subjects of interest covered by guest speakers might include those pertaining to the diet practices of thyroid patients, partnering with their doctors, best methods for taking their medications and any other subject of interest for the group, to help better inform them.

Providing an Online Forum

A support group administrator might also choose to create an accompanying forum for members who may wish to communicate between meetings or might actually choose to create the support group as a whole, as an online resource. A forum requires a degree of moderation, so that unwanted posts or spam can be deleted or edited. The forum could also be restricted to those who are members of the support group. A forum can be a great resource of ongoing communication, for added support and shared information.

The forum moderator(s) would also want to put effort into making sure the forum stays on-subject for each topic-category that might be included in the forum and to make sure small offshoots of members are not formed which can sometimes evolve into exclusionary cliques. Any hurtful practices would also need to be addressed such as gossip or posts that degrade into personal attacks. If these types of things are closely moderated, a forum can be an excellent resource for thyroid disease patients and some online hosts make forums available free of charge.

CHAPTER SIXTEEN

Thyroid Disease Related Digestive Disorders

Bowel Function Problems and Indigestion

Patients with either hypothyroidism or hyperthyroidism can experience symptoms related to their digestive tracts that improve with treatment of thyroid hormone imbalance.

An under active thyroid gland or "hypothyroidism" causes a decrease in bodily metabolism which affects the rate at which digestion occurs, resulting in symptoms related to slowed bowel movements and digestion. With overactive thyroid conditions or "hyperthyroidism" metabolism is sped-up, causing an abnormal increase in the rate of digestion and bowel activity. The goal of treatment for both types of thyroid disorders is to correct the metabolism back to a normal level by either replacing low levels of thyroid hormones or by slowing down the over-production of them.

Constipation

With hypothyroidism, foods are converted into fuels for energy in the body at a slower rate than in people with normal metabolisms. This can cause bowel movements to be less-frequent and can cause them to become hardened and dryer than normal. A build up in the bowels can also occur causing discomfort, bloating and pain in the stomach and painful bowel movements.

In some cases of autoimmune hypothyroidism called "Hashimoto's thyroiditis", when intermittent phases of hyperthyroidism also occur (Hashitoxicosis), a person can alternate between spells of constipation and diarrhea. If thyroid disease is not diagnosed, the person may believe the condition is caused by IBS (Irritable Bowel Syndrome).

Diarrhea

People with hyperthyroid conditions, will commonly experience chronic diarrhea (ongoing and severe). This is due to the body rapidly converting foods into fuel or what is also referred to as "metabolic energy", faster than with normal metabolism. Foods will quickly move through the digestive tract, causing frequent, loose or runny bowel movements.

In addition to symptoms of stomach cramping and the need to make emergency trips to the bathroom, frequent diarrhea can also cause dehydration and essential nutrients to not be fully absorbed into the body, which can lead to malnutrition if treatment for hyperthyroidism is delayed.

Indigestion

Medical sources state that both underproduction and overproduction of stomach acid can cause symptoms of heartburn, sour stomach and acid reflux. With hyperthyroid conditions when stomach acid levels rise to abnormally high levels (hyperchlorhydria) due to increased digestion, heartburn symptoms can occur commonly.

Patients who have not received a diagnosis of thyroid disorder may instead be diagnosed with common acid reflux or with the more severe digestive disorder called Gastroesophageal Reflux Disease (GERD). The same is true of hypothyroid conditions, in which there can be a lack of stomach acid available to digest foods at a normal rate (hypochlorhydria).

Treatments

In most cases of digestive problems caused by thyroid disorders, bringing thyroid hormone levels back into normal range will significantly reduce or eliminate symptoms. If symptoms persist following treatment, over-the-counter or prescription medications for indigestion symptoms or irregular bowel movements may be needed.

In addition to drug treatments, there are lifestyle and diet methods that can also help. These include eating smaller meals and consuming them slowly, eliminating use of stimulants such as alcohol, coffee and tobacco, reducing stress, not eating for two hours before bedtime and elevating the head of the bed or sleeping on an extra pillow to prevent acid reflux.

Constipation can be helped by eating foods rich in fiber, four hours apart from thyroid hormone dose, including fruits, vegetables and legumes (beans, lentils, and peanuts) and drinking plenty of water (approximately 64oz per day). Stubborn diarrhea symptoms can be additionally helped by avoiding high-fiber in the diet and foods that are greasy or that contain high levels of diary or refined sugars,

CHAPTER SEVENTEEN

Symptoms Associated with Thyroid Autoimmunity

Problems Not Directly Related to Hormone Levels

In addition to symptoms that occur due to thyroid hormone imbalances, they may also occur as a result of autoimmune thyroid disease processes.

According to a number of studies published on the PubMed (U.S. National Institutes of Health) website and other medical sources, thyroid autoimmunity can contribute to a variety of symptom-manifestations in patients whose thyroid hormone levels have not yet fallen outside of normal values. Symptoms to varied degrees may also continue to occur in patients whose thyroid hormone imbalances have been corrected.

Goiter and Thyroid Nodules

In some cases of autoimmune thyroid diseases, a mild goiter (thyroid enlargement) is the first symptom that manifests. This can be true of both Hashimoto's thyroiditis (autoimmune hypothyroidism) and Graves' disease (autoimmune hyperthyroidism). The goiter can appear in advance of abnormal thyroid hormone levels, resulting from inflammation in the gland rather than directly resulting from thyroid hormone imbalance. The same is true of thyroid nodules (small tumor-like growths) which can develop in thyroid glands with abnormal tissue in them caused by thyroid autoimmunity but that have not yet begun to dysfunction in producing thyroid hormones.

Anxiety and Mood Disorders

According to Dr. Richard C. W. Hall, MD, a medical researcher for Johns Hopkins University and a forensic psychiatrist, anxiety symptoms can be the first to manifest in patients with Hashimoto's thyroiditis, the autoimmune cause of hypothyroidism. In his article titled "Anxiety and Endocrine Disease", he states that anxiety can be the prominent and initial symptom observed in newly diagnosed Hashimoto's patients.

Other research articles address the association of mood and anxiety disorders with thyroid autoimmunity, including one titled "A case control study on psychiatric disorders in Hashimoto disease and euthyroid goiter: not only depressive but also anxiety disorders are associated with thyroid autoimmunity". The research conclusion in this study states that these psychiatric manifestations occur in some patients, independent of thyroid hormone levels, meaning they are not directly caused by thyroid hormone imbalance but caused by the auto-antibodies that are present in thyroid diseases.

Rheumatic Symptoms

In a PubMed published medical research article titled "Chronic autoimmune thyroiditis and rheumatic manifestations." the study concludes that rheumatic symptoms, meaning those affecting muscles and joints can occur in patients with Hashimoto's thyroiditis due to the thyroid autoimmunity and not a direct result of abnormal thyroid hormone levels. The article goes on to state that the joint and muscles aches and stiffness (rheumatic symptoms) can occur in some euthyroid patients which are those whose thyroid hormone levels fall within normal values.

Chronic Fatigue

In another medical research study, published by Alan R. Gaby, M.D., patients with Chronic Fatigue Syndrome (CFS) were blood tested for thyroid autoimmunity but a significant percent of them were found to be negative for thyroid disease causing auto-antibodies. Upon performing a Fine Needle Aspiration on these same CFS patients, it was revealed that 40% of them were experiencing chronic lymphocytic thyroiditis (Hashimoto's) but were not yet manifesting abnormal thyroid hormone levels detectable by blood lab testing.

Symptoms of thyroid autoimmunity can range from mild to moderate as described in the preceding subheadings or can become severe and even life-threatening as can occur in a rare condition called "Hashimoto's Encephalopathy".

While it is widely believed that thyroid disease symptoms only begin to appear in patients when thyroid hormone levels become imbalanced, the above cited research studies indicate that symptoms can manifest in advance of hormone imbalance, resulting instead from the autoimmune disease process.

CHAPTER EIGHTEEN

Thyroid Disease and Neuropathy Symptoms

Neurological Problems in Hypothyroid and Hyperthyroid Patients

Thyroid disease can present with symptoms of peripheral

neuropathy and other neurological problems, which may not fully resolve with hormone treatment in all patients.

The thyroid hormone imbalances caused by thyroid diseases are an obvious cause of neurological symptoms but what role does "thyroid autoimmunity" play in these type symptoms? Autoimmune-caused hypothyroidism is called Hashimoto's thyroiditis and autoimmune-caused hyperthyroidism is called Graves' disease. Medical research conclusions on studies of thyroid patients has shown that the disease process itself may contribute to neurological symptoms in some thyroid patients in spite of correcting abnormal thyroid hormone levels.

Thyroid Related Neuropathy Symptoms

Neuropathy symptoms include those having to do with nerve functions throughout the body. Common neurological symptoms include headaches, numbness or tingling in the hands and/or feet (peripheral neuropathy), abnormal reflexes and muscle weakness and spasms. Thyroid disease is an endocrine gland disorder (hormone related) and all disorders in this category, including diabetes have potential to cause neurological symptoms. In the case of thyroid disease, the hormones produced by this endocrine gland regulate the metabolism in every cell of the body, including those related to nerve function. When a disorder affecting thyroid hormone balance develops, the function of the nervous system can be sped-up or slowed down, resulting in nerve-related symptoms.

Treating Thyroid Hormone Imbalances

Hypothyroidism is a condition in which thyroid hormone levels drop below normal. This results in all bodily functions slowing down (hypo-metabolism), including brain-nerve signals (motor responses). It also causes fluid build up in tissues of the body or what is referred to as "myxedema", which can cause pressure on nerves, resulting in additional symptoms of neuropathy, such as numbness and tingling in the extremities. When thyroid hormones are brought back up to correct levels, these type symptoms improve, as well as myxedema in body tissues affecting nerve signals.

Hyperthyroidism is a condition of abnormally high thyroid hormone levels, which causes all bodily functions to become sped up (hyper-metabolism). Muscle reflexes are hyper-reactive, meaning there is abnormal muscle tension in response to brain-nerve signals. This can result in the adverse effect following physical activity, of severe muscle weakness. Some patients may also experience episodes of muscle paralysis and/or muscle deterioration. Neurological symptoms that accompany hyperthyroid conditions are sometimes referred to as "thyrotoxic myopathy" but will improve significantly with treatment to reduce thyroid hormone levels and treatment for symptoms of an overactive metabolism via anti-thyroid drugs and beta-blockers.

Thyroid Antibodies

For those patients whose neuropathies do not fully resolve with treatment for thyroid hormone imbalance, another factor in causing symptoms that should be considered is the disease process of thyroid autoimmunity itself. The auto-antibodies sent from the immune system to attack the thyroid gland may also exert negative effects on the peripheral nervous system. Some of this may be the result of inflammation in the body that begins to effect nerve function. With "Hashimoto's Encephalopathy" for example, which can result from Hashimoto's thyroiditis in very rare cases, severe and even life-threatening neurological symptoms can develop. It would seem obvious that neuropathies may manifest in Hashimoto's patients to lesser degrees as well.

Other medical research studies have found that some autoimmune thyroid disease patients have other auto-antibodies present as well, that can directly affect the nervous system. This includes studies that have found mild manifestations of other autoimmune diseases present in thyroid patients including symptoms of Myasthenia Gravis. There is no cure for auto-antibodies but keeping thyroid hormone disorders well-treated can help and some research suggests that supplementing patients with selenium may help to reduce thyroid antibody levels. Anti-inflammatory medications can also help in patients with highly elevated inflammation levels.

CHAPTER NINTEEN

Thyroid Disease and Chronic Fatigue Syndrome

Misdiagnosis and Co-morbid Diagnosis

Thyroid disease has many of the same symptoms as Chronic Fatigue Syndrome and in fact the two conditions can coexist or in some cases have been misdiagnosed.

When these two conditions have been misdiagnosed (confused) it is mostly due to early onset thyroid disease being elusive to diagnostic blood testing. Most cases of thyroid hormone imbalance in industrialized countries are caused by an autoimmune process in which the thyroid gland experiences slow destruction from auto-antibodies attacking it. In some cases, these antibodies are not detected in the blood despite the fact that they are present and causing the disease process that eventually leads to hypothyroidism (under-active thyroid).

Hashimoto's Thyroiditis

This autoimmune cause of hypothyroidism, also referred to as chronic lymphocytic thyroiditis, sometimes requires a tissue biopsy called an "FNA" (Fine Needle Aspiration) to be detected. This is a procedure whereby a local anesthesia is administered to the patient so that a hypodermic needle designed to extract a tissue sample from the thyroid gland can be inserted. Analysis is then performed on the sample to determine if thyroid disease is present or to help rule it out as the problem causing symptoms in a patient.

In an article authored by Alan R. Gaby, M.D. (B.A. from Yale University, M.S. in biochemistry from Emory University, and his M.D. from the University of Maryland.) that is titled "Autoimmune thyroiditis as a cause of chronic fatigue", he details a medical research study involving 219 patients with Chronic Fatigue Syndrome (CFS), having severe fatigue of at least 1-year in duration. While only half of the patients were found positive for either antithyroidperoxidase antibodies (Anti-TPO) or antithyroglobulin antibodies (Anti-TG), 40% were found to have definite histological evidence of Hashimoto's thyroiditis.

Hypothyroidism Elusive to TSH Testing

The study-patients in the research cited by Dr. Gaby MD, had varied TSH readings upon being blood tested (pituitary hormone that reflects thyroid hormone levels) with many falling within normal lab values. The study points out that possibly up to 40% of CFS patients are experiencing thyroid disease that will be responsive to thyroid hormone replacement therapy and that hypothyroidism causing symptoms, can be present despite normal TSH levels. It also points out that FNA may be required to detect autoimmune thyroiditis in a significant number of cases.

U.S./NIH Says CFS Can Co-Exist With Thyroid Disease

In previous years, before more research was conducted on the association of thyroid disease to CFS, it was stated by reputable medical entities including the Centers for Disease Control (U.S. National Institutes of Health), that a diagnosis of an endocrine disorder or disease, including that affecting thyroid function, would rule-out a diagnosis of CFS. This stance has changed however in recent years, with these same medical sources now stating that CFS can be co-morbid (co-existing) with these other types of health disorders.

It is further believed by other medical research groups that autoimmune and endocrine disease may actually serve as triggers for the development of syndromes such as CFS and fibromyalgia. Research continues in attempt to find more answers to these complicated and sometimes mysterious health disorders.

CHAPTER TWENTY

Home Thyroid Function Tests

Are They Reliable?

Thyroid disease diagnosis must come through a licensed medical practitioner. There are, however tests that can be done at home to help identify thyroid problems.

A person who suspects he may have a thyroid disease or disorder should never attempt to self-diagnose because there are medical conditions that can have similar symptoms. While this is an important fact to consider, there are also things a person can do to help monitor his body for signs and symptoms that might point to a thyroid problem.

Patients can add any findings via these tests to their discussion with a qualified MD, who can make a definitive diagnosis through additional testing or rule-out thyroid issues as being the problem. The following subheadings list three areas of self-tests or observations that can aid in reports a patient relates to his doctor. Some may be more reliable than others but none of them are harmful or dangerous and may actually help to identify thyroid-related problems in some cases.

Iodine Spot Test

Some medical sources have stated that a drop of iodine placed on an area of soft skin on the body and then observed to see how quickly it is absorbed, can help indicate how well the thyroid is functioning. A product with high iodine content is suggested for this test, such as the "Lugol's Solution" brand that leaves a goldish colored spot on the skin when a drop is placed on the inside of the upper arm.

If a drop of iodine placed on the skin absorbs (disappears) within an hour or two rather than remaining for approximately 18 hours, this may indicate that the thyroid is lacking enough healthy tissue within it to absorb an adequate amount of iodine from foods eaten. The body responds by immediately sending any iodine in the body to the gland, in attempt to increase thyroid function. The test may also help indicate when hypothyroidism is caused by iodine deficiency.

Observing Myxedema

This condition associated with both hypothyroidism and hyperthyroidism, causes fluid to build in tissues of the body. The term was used to also describe the overall symptoms of hypothyroidism for many years, going back to the earliest days of diagnosing thyroid disorders. It is most commonly found in patients with Hashimoto's thyroiditis, the autoimmune cause of hypothyroidism. Rather than simply being water retention, the tissues will actually begin to expand due to increase of mucus in the membranes and damage to tissues and scarring of them can occur in some cases.

This reaction in the body, to thyroid hormone imbalance, causes a puffy appearance in the face and will also cause areas of the body to have a thicker texture to them which can sometimes be felt by lightly pinching soft areas of the epidermis (deep skin areas), such as the outside of the upper arms. It can sometimes also be detected by pressing these areas of the skin with a fingertip for a few seconds and seeing if it leaves a yellowish mark or an indentation on the skin. The most obvious way to detect myxedema however is by simply observing any signs of swelling in the body that will be most obvious in the face and in the extremities (legs and arms).

Monitoring Basal Body Temperature

This method for detecting low body temperature which can be somewhat subtle in mild to moderate hypothyroid conditions, requires checking it upon first waking in the morning using a basal body thermometer (BBT). This type is different from typical temperature types used to detect fever and have a different normal range and measurement intervals on them for detecting very mild body temperature changes. Abnormally low body temperature can be one indicator of a slowed metabolism caused by a lack of thyroid hormone in the body.

Basal thermometers are used to help determine times of earliest ovulation in women attempting pregnancy but who are experiencing fertility problems of their own or that of their spouses and the best time for impregnation is being determined. They can also help detect abnormal body temperatures in people experiencing thyroid hormone imbalances. Earliest wake-time readings are taken for several mornings and the temperatures are recorded to see if below-normal, borderline-low or low-normal readings occur, indicating possible hypothyroidism.

Diagnosis Comes Through Qualified Physicians

Before the advent of thyroid blood testing, the basal body temperature method and observing patients for signs of myxedema were used often in helping determine metabolic problems in the body caused by thyroid dysfunction. One medical researcher who became well-known for these methods was Professor Broda O. Barnes MD, whose research is being continued to this day at a research institute named after him. None of these methods addressed above should replace diagnosis by a qualified doctor and should simply be viewed as preliminary methods, with blood testing and other diagnostic tests being those that obtain definitive diagnoses.

CHAPTER TWENTYONE

Goiter and Thyroid Nodule Self-Examination

Palpating and Observing the Gland for Abnormalities

While a person can sometimes detect a goiter and/or thyroid nodules by self examination, a definitive diagnoses must be given by a qualified physician.

These abnormalities in size and/or texture of the thyroid gland can occur with both hypothyroid and hyperthyroid conditions but are more common in autoimmune thyroid diseases. If a person feels he may be experiencing thyroid-related symptoms or has detected an abnormal feeling in his thyroid, a preliminary self-examination can be done while an appointment with a qualified physician has been scheduled.

A patient can then report any findings that indicate problems in the gland to his medical doctor. The emedicine/WebMD website states in their article titled "Goiter Nontoxic: Follow-Up", under the Patient Education sub-heading that "Thyroid self-examination" may be taught to patients, allowing them to monitor their own body for early changes in gland size."

Palpating the Thyroid Gland

A person can feel his own throat, using the fingertips (palpation), in the area of the thyroid gland, to detect swelling or lumps. The thyroid is located in the center of the throat, directly beneath the Adams apple, which in males is more prominent but can usually be located easily in females as well. Once finding the Adams apple, the isthmus (middle portion) of the thyroid is only about an inch or, slightly lower below it and will be slightly raised. If the isthmus protrudes significantly, or feels very firm to the touch, this can indicate a goiter in that portion of the gland.

Shape of the Gland

There are also two lobes of the thyroid gland, one of each side of it, that extend about an inch toward the inside of the throat and that extend upward toward the Adams apple, about even with it. The gland is typically small and forms a butterfly shape. The lobes actually attach to the Adams apple and throat with connecting cartilage and tissue but when they are normal size, are usually not easily felt unless pressed-on firmly with the fingertips. If they are easily detectable without firmly pressing down on them or are visible without the need to palpate them, this can indicate a goiter or nodules in the lobe-areas as well.

The Swallow Test

While palpation is being done to detect swelling (enlargement) in the gland, any lumps or protrusions that might indicate a thyroid nodule (tumor-like growth) or several of them should also be checked for. These can also be spotted by tilting the head back, while looking in a mirror and taking sips of water, watching for any signs of enlargement or lumps as the gland moves up and down in the throat. Some people with enlarged glands are found to have both goiter and nodules, which is referred to as a "nodular goiter" or a "multi-nodular goiter".

Difficulty Swallowing

If a person feels a lump on the inside of his throat when swallowing, this can indicate a thyroid nodule that is growing toward the inside and that cannot be felt from the outside of the throat. If there is a general feeling of difficulty swallowing or breathing due to the throat being constricted, this may also indicate a goiter in which the enlargement is swelling toward the inside of the throat. This type problem is not always indicative of thyroid problems but can be related to esophagus problems as well.

If any of these self-examination methods are found to indicate a problem in the gland, it should be reported to a medical doctor as soon as possible for further evaluation.

CHAPTER TWENTYTWO

SSRI Antidepressants for Thyroid Patients

When Hormone Therapy Does Not Improve Emotional Symptoms

Patients who have been well-treated for either hypothyroidism or hyperthyroidism may sometimes need the additional help of SSRI antidepressant medications.

Getting thyroid hormones back into balance when the thyroid is overactive or under-active can go a long way toward relieving symptoms of anxiety and/or depression. For some thyroid patients however, emotional symptoms will linger even after adequate or optimal treatment is administered for their thyroid disorder. SSRI antidepressants are often the treatment that is added to address stubborn emotional symptoms.

Emotional Symptoms Associated With Thyroid Autoimmunity

According to medical research published on the PubMed website (U.S. Gov.-National Institutes of Health), anxiety and mood disorders can be directly related to "anti-thyroidperoxidase auto-antibodies" (anti-TPO). These are the antibodies found in most cases of thyroid diseases caused by an immune system response, in which they are sent to attack protein/enzymes in the thyroid gland.

One particular study entitled "The link between thyroid autoimmunity (antithyroid peroxidase autoantibodies) with anxiety and mood disorders in the community: a field of interest for public health in the future", states that psychiatric disorders in thyroid patients may be rooted in the "thyroid autoimmunity" and not easily correctable. There are a number of other studies with similar conclusions. These type studies demonstrate the fact that correcting thyroid hormone imbalances does not treat or halt the disease process itself and therefore symptoms such as the emotional ones may need additional treatments.

SSRI Antidepressants Can Decrease Thyroid Hormones

SSRI stands for "selective serotonin reuptake inhibitors"

and is the most commonly prescribed type of antidepressant, for both anxiety and depression symptoms. Medical research studies have found that SSRI antidepressants can cause a slight decrease in both the T3 and T4 thyroid hormone levels. In one study, this conclusion came after trials of the drug were given to 19 patients with major depression and their blood baseline thyroid hormone levels before the trial were compared to their retested levels following the drug treatment and post-treatment levels were significantly lowered by the drug.

The research study titled "Peripheral thyroid hormones and response to selective serotonin reuptake inhibitors" also mentions the fact that keeping thyroid hormone levels at "optimal" range in patients treated with SSRI drugs can increase the effectiveness of antidepressant treatment. This is mentioned despite the fact that the participants used in the drug trial were not thyroid patients. This would seem to indicate even more importance in treated thyroid patients having optimal thyroid hormone levels to aid in SSRI antidepressant treatment.

Adjusting the Thyroid Hormone Therapy Dose

With the fact that an SSRI drug may decrease a treated hypothyroid patient's thyroid hormone levels, a treating doctor may want to retest a patient being treated with the drug, to see what hormone dose adjustments might be needed. If a patient has been on thyroid hormone therapy long enough to only require blood retesting of their hormone levels every three to six months, adding an SSRI antidepressant might require that the blood retest scheduling be shortened.

The blood retesting typically used in newly treated hypothyroid patients, which would be about every 8-weeks, might be a good idea until an antidepressant has also fully adjusted in the body. This way the doctor can see if the drug has any lowering affect on thyroid hormone levels, so that they can be raised accordingly. Optimizing treatment for hypothyroidism may lend toward greater success in treating emotional symptoms with SSRI antidepressants.

CHAPTER TWENTYTHREE

Famous Men and Women with Thyroid Disease

Celebrities with Hypothyroid and Hyperthyroid Disorders

Many famous people have come forward to relate the fact that they suffer various thyroid conditions. Their stories have helped educate the public about these diseases.

When celebrities share the details of their battles with thyroid disorders, this brings more awareness to the general public about symptoms and diagnosis of hypothyroid and hyperthyroid conditions. Some have also gone public with their stories about diagnosed thyroid cancers they have been treated for which also helps bring more attention to cancer awareness.

Oprah Winfrey

One of the celebrity stories that have helped gain public exposure for thyroid disease in recent years is that of Oprah Winfrey. In the year 2007, Oprah announced her diagnosis including details about her symptom struggles that had plagued her for years previous but that had worsened during months previous to her diagnosis. While she did not specify that her thyroid disease is autoimmune in nature, meaning the immune system creating antibodies to attack the thyroid gland, she did state that her body had "turned against itself".

In her descriptions of symptoms experienced, she mentioned going through anxiety and sleeplessness for weeks at a time and having experienced a panic attack at one point. Her hyperthyroid (overactive) type symptoms were followed by a period of severe fatigue and the need to sleep more hours than normal, plus her weight-gain began to escalate rapidly. This description sounds very much like the symptom phases, patients with Hashimoto's thyroiditis go through (autoimmune hypothyroidism, first manifesting as hyperthyroidism) and many who have watched this story unfold believe this to be the disease she has.

Observers of Oprah at the time noticed she was looking ill and very tired and in the mean time she was trying to find out what was wrong with her, which required seeing several doctors before one recommended thyroid blood testing. Her hypothyroidism was revealed on test results and she is now being treated, although her treatment does not sound conventional, with her recent mentions of not being required to take thyroid hormone replacement therapy. The world continues to watch for any new developments in Oprah's case.

Professional Athletes

Both male and female athletes have gone public with their thyroid disease stories. Two track and field gold medal winners have been treated for thyroid disorders including

Gail Devers, a 3-time female Olympic gold winner in the 100 meter hurdles and Carl Lewis, a male competitor who has won many gold medals, including the top spot for 10 years consecutively in the Olympic long jump. Two other male professional athletes that have come forward with thyroid disease diagnoses include Bobby Ingram NFL, wide receiver for the Seattle Seahawks, and professional golfer Ben Crenshaw who has won the PGA championship, the Masters and the British Open.

Presidents, Comedians and Artists

President George H. W. Bush, the 41st U.S. President suffered Graves' disease (autoimmune hyperthyroidism) for which he was treated and is now taking thyroid hormone replacement therapy to treat resulting hypothyroidism. His first symptoms were atrial fibrillation, severe fatigue, hand-tremors and a mild goiter. Amazingly, President Bush's wife Barbara and his dog Millie were also diagnosed with diseases causing them hyperthyroidism. It is believed that the second U.S. President, John Adams also suffered from Graves' disease-hyperthyroidism.

Italian comedian and actor Joe Piscopo was diagnosed and treated for thyroid cancer in 1990 and has been in full remission since. Other artists in various fields of media and art have been diagnosed with thyroid disorders, including musician Rod Stewart, movie critic Roger Ebert and cowboy artist Charles M. Russell. All of these individuals from so many fields of endeavor, demonstrate the fact that thyroid disease is not selective about whom it affects.

CHAPTER TWENTYFOUR

Diagnosing Benign and Malignant Thyroid Nodules

Suspicious and Non-Suspicious Tumors in the Gland

Thyroid nodules are tumor-like growths that can develop within the thyroid gland and can vary in size, texture and ability to change thyroid hormone levels.

Some medical estimates state that up to 10% of the general population has thyroid nodules that are detectable by feel (fingertip-palpation), while autopsy studies have revealed that up to 50% of the population has them. Most thyroid nodules do not pose a problem, while others cause difficulty with swallowing or breathing and others cause an imbalance in thyroid hormone levels.

Even less common are thyroid nodules that contain cancer cells or "malignancy" but most are benign, meaning they are not cancerous. Malignant thyroid nodules are diagnosed more often in women than in men and are also found more often in younger patients under the age of 20-years and older patients at the age of 70-years and older.

Common Vs Suspicious Nodules

The most commonly detected thyroid nodules in the general population are those that are not solid but contain fluid within them, giving them a soft texture or what are sometimes referred to as "cystic nodules". These types do not pose a risk of containing malignancy, the vast majority of the time and so are usually not referred for additional testing beyond palpation to determine their size and texture.

Having a number of nodules in one's thyroid gland (multi-nodular), rather than a singular one also helps to rule out the possibility of thyroid cancer. Lone thyroid nodules and those that are very firm in texture are often referred for additional testing that might include tissue biopsy and/or imaging tests.

Hot Nodules

This term is used to describe thyroid nodules that begin to act like normal thyroid tissue, meaning they absorb iodine and begin producing thyroid hormone as if they are part of the gland. A nuclear imaging scan, followed by oral or intravenous dosing of a patient with radioactive iodine, will show that the nodule is a "hot area" on the scan which means it is absorbing large amounts of iodine within the thyroid gland. These types are rarely suspicious of containing malignancy but often cause hyperthyroidism in patients who have them. This may require surgical removal of the nodule and or part or all of the thyroid gland.

Solid Cold Nodules and Malignancy

These types have a firm texture when palpated and may be found singular or less-commonly within a group of nodules. These, type can take up space in the thyroid gland and cause a degree of hypothyroidism, meaning slowed production of thyroid hormone. They are often also of significant size that presents more concern, which would be in the 3-centimeter and larger category.

Even if nodules are smaller but are of solid texture, they are often referred for imaging scans. This might include an MRI scan with contrast, a thyroid ultrasound or a Radionuclide Scan in which a dose of "radioactive iodine isotope-123" is administered to a patient, followed by taking images with a nuclear camera.

If a nodule shows up as a "cold area" on the test result, meaning an area that appears blank because it did not absorb the radioactive iodine, this can indicate malignancy and the patient would likely be referred for thyroid removal. The tumor/nodule would either require removal of the affected lobe, referred to as a "lobectomy" or "partial thyroidectomy" (sub-total) but more commonly will require total thyroidectomy, followed by radiation treatment to eradicate any remaining cancer cells.

The patient would afterward require thyroid hormone replacement due to the missing thyroid gland and resulting hypothyroidism but hormone therapy may be delayed for weeks following completion of radiation treatments. The most common malignancies found in thyroid nodules, are papillary, follicular, medullary and anaplastic (most radical type) cancers.

Tissue Biopsies

In some cases the diagnostic tests for detecting or ruling-out malignant cells in thyroid nodules are tissue biopsies. Some nodules require surgical biopsy, if they are found growing toward the inside of the throat but most are detectable from the outside of the throat. These can be biopsied by "Fine-Needle Aspiration", a test using a long hypodermic needle, inserted into the neck to extract a tissue sample after the patient is given a local anesthesia. The sample is then analyzed for detection of any suspicious cells.

CHAPTER TWENTYFIVE

Common Primary and Secondary Causes of Goiters

Typical Conditions That Result in Thyroid Enlargement

A goiter means that the thyroid gland has become enlarged. Goiters can have primary or secondary causes or may have no apparent cause.

The mid-portion of the thyroid gland or the "isthmus" is located in the center of the neck, below the Adam's apple and has two lobes on each side of it, creating a butterfly shape. Under certain circumstances, the isthmus and/or one or both of the lobes can become enlarged. Enlargement is not always accompanied by inflammation in the gland or caused by a disease process within the gland.

Nontoxic Typical Diffuse Goiter

This type of goiter, also called a "simple goiter" can have a primary or secondary cause and is not toxic, meaning it is one that does not cause the gland to release excessive hormone causing hyperthyroidism (abnormally high levels). These type goiters can manifest without explanation or may be the result of thyroid autoimmunity (primary) or types of temporary viral thyroiditis and pregnancy (secondary causes). These type goiters cause enlargement in the gland not due to thyroid nodules (tumorous growths). Cases of this type goiter that have no obvious explanation may not lead to thyroid hormone imbalance of any kind.

Endemic Goiters

This type of secondary goiter, which can also be referred to as a "colloid goiter" is caused by iodine deficiency which means low levels of iodine are resulting in swelling of the gland and is not a problem or disease within the gland itself. This type goiter is common in third world countries where diets are poor in iodine content and where table salt is not iodized. Some endemic goiters are also found to contain thyroid nodules (small tumors) within them, which is called a "colloid nodular goiter".

Toxic Diffuse Goiter

This term is in reference to a primary goiter that directly causes hyperthyroidism. The "diffuse" aspect of the term is reference to the fact that toxic thyroid nodules are not what are causing the hyperthyroidism or the sole reason for the gland-swelling although nodules may also be present. This term is often used synonymously with Graves' disease.

Multi-nodular Goiter

This type goiter is primary because it is a problem within the gland itself and results from accumulation of several (multi) nodules within the gland. There may be swelling within the gland itself, as well but if the thyroid is enlarged due to the nodules alone, the term for the condition remains the same. If any of the nodules are hormone producing or "hot", the term for the condition would be "Toxic Multi-Nodular Goiter". This type goiter can be present in Graves' disease patients as well as in Hashimoto's thyroiditis patients but the later autoimmune condition (Hashimoto's) would not present with permanent, progressive hyperthyroidism as Graves' does.

Treatment for Goiters

Treatments vary according to the cause of the goiter. If iodine deficiency is the cause, replacing this essential element to bring it back to adequate levels will resolve the problem. If a goiter is caused by thyroid hormone imbalance, correcting these levels back to normal values can help resolve the condition and can aid in shrinking both goiters and thyroid nodules. If goiters are large enough to pose a danger of hindering a patient's breathing or swallowing, partial or total thyroid removal by surgical thyroidectomy or radioactive iodine ablation might be the procedures that are ordered.

Some goiters are not typical but have uncommon aspects to them and in these cases may require special treatments. In cases where severe hyperthyroidism is present, beta-blockers and anti-thyroid drugs may also be administered and anti-inflammatory drugs, in the case of severe inflammation. Following some of these procedures, patients may become hypothyroid and will require life-long thyroid hormone replacement therapy afterward.

CHAPTER TWENTYSIX

Rare Causes of Thyroid Gland Enlargement

Uncommon Conditions that Cause Goiters

The vast majority of enlarged thyroid glands occur due to common diseases or conditions but there are cases in which goiters do not have typical causes.

The most common cause of goiter worldwide is iodine deficiency with thyroid autoimmunity being the second major cause, the class of thyroid disease that presents with auto-antibodies attacking the thyroid gland. The two resulting autoimmune disorders that often present with goiters are Graves' disease which results in hyperthyroidism and Hashimoto's thyroiditis which results in hypothyroidism. There are less common causes of goiters as well and some of these will be addressed in the following subheadings.

Uncommon Sporadic Goiter

This type of primary goiter (a problem within the gland) is also sometimes placed in the "simple goiter" category, meaning there is enlargement without actual development of abnormal thyroid tissue and is commonly an inherited genetic condition. Some cases of sporadic goiters however, also include those in which diseased thyroid tissue grows outside of the normal boundaries of the gland. This can include thyroid autoimmunity diseases, thyroid nodules and a less common type of condition called Riedel's thyroiditis. This latter mentioned disease causes thyroid tissue to be replaced with fibrous tissue that can grow large enough to obstruct breathing and swallowing. This overgrowth of the thyroid gland can also occur with types of thyroid cancer, including papillary, follicular and sarcomatoid carcinomas.

Exophthalmic Goiter

This type of goiter that can be either primary or secondary (indirectly affecting the gland) manifests with severe hyperthyroidism and with a condition of protruding eyeballs or "proptosis" (a type of Thyroid Eye Disease). The term for this type goiter can also be synonymous with

Grave's disease (primary) but rarely the condition can be caused by a shortage of necessary enzymes in the thyroid that allows toxins to build within the gland. Some medical sources believe the condition may rarely also result from chronic alcohol abuse (secondary).

Severe and even life-threatening symptoms including hypertension, tachycardia (rapid heart rate) and other heart arrhythmias can occur with this condition. Some cases may be caused by brain lesions (secondary) that disrupt the manufacture of key thyroid enzymes. In this case it would not be caused by thyroid autoimmunity as Grave's disease is. This rare, severe version of the disorder can be fatal if treatment with beta-blockers to regulate blood pressure and cardiac symptoms is not administered. Patients may also be referred for emergency thyroid removal (surgical thyroidectomy).

Congenital Goiter

If a baby is born with thyroid swelling, this term for the primary goiter is used. The goiter may be accompanied by hypothyroidism in the newborn as well, which is referred to as congenital hypothyroidism but some of them manifest without thyroid hormone imbalance or may occur with mild hypothyroidism. If thyroid nodules are also present, it is referred to as Congenital Nodular Goiter. Most cases of this type goiter are temporary and only require short-term treatment to resolve them.

Diagnosis and Treatment

Goiters, regardless of cause have treatments available for them, depending on the manifestations and the symptoms that may accompany them. If a person detects swelling or lumps in their thyroid gland, which is located at the front of the neck just below the Adams apple area, they should report to their doctor for further evaluation. A doctor will often first palpate the gland, meaning to examine it by feel using the fingertips and may also order diagnostic imaging tests and/or tissue biopsy. Blood tests of thyroid hormone levels and/or to detect thyroid antibodies may also be ordered to help determine the cause and treatments that are needed for common goiters and for those that are less typical.

CHAPTER TWENTYSEVEN

Conditions that Merit Thyroid Removal

When should the Gland be Removed?

There are a number of conditions that may result in a treating doctor referring a patient for thyroidectomy or radioactive iodine ablation of the thyroid gland.

Doctors usually recommend thyroid removal as a last resort due to risks that are involved with any type of surgery or procedure involving major organs or glands in the body. The thyroid gland is a major metabolism-regulating endocrine gland and it has four parathyroid glands sitting on the posterior surface (behind it) that regulate calcium levels in the body. It is also due to risk of damage to the parathyroid glands that thyroid removal is only recommended when it is absolutely necessary.

Thyroid Cancer

When suspicious, abnormal tissue in the thyroid gland is detected or there is a nodule (tumor) in the gland that is of significant size or of solid texture, a tissue biopsy called an FNA – Fine Needle Aspiration or surgical biopsy will be ordered. If malignant cells are found, in most cases, a total thyroidectomy will be ordered. If suspicion of cancer is only found in a nodule affecting one lobe of the thyroid, only that side of the gland may be removed.

This is referred to as a sub-total thyroidectomy or a lobectomy, depending on how much of the gland is removed. Once partial or full removal has been completed, the patient may then undergo ionizing radiation therapy to destroy any remaining cancer cells that might be left behind. Afterward, any lowering of thyroid hormone levels will be replaced with thyroid hormone replacement therapy but may not be administered until all radiation treatments are completed and time is given for radiation levels to diminish from the body.

Goiters and Nodules

If a patient has a large goiter, meaning thyroid-swelling, a treating doctor may first attempt to shrink the thyroid by administering thyroid hormone therapy. If this is not successful in reducing the goiter or if the gland has already grown to a size that places the patient at danger of having difficulty breathing or swallowing, a thyroidectomy might be recommended. This is also true of thyroid nodules that can begin to grow on the inside of the gland that is nearest the esophagus and that are not palpable (able to be felt) or visible from the outside.

These can become large enough to obstruct breathing or swallowing and may result in the need for partial of full thyroid removal, even if there is no suspicion for malignancy in the nodule. A combination of thyroid nodules with goiter can also cause problems in some patients if it causes significant enlargement, which is referred to as a multi-nodular goiter. Thyroid hormone replacement may be necessary following thyroid removal for these reasons as well.

Widely Fluctuating Thyroid Hormone Levels

While it is not common, there are patients with thyroid autoimmunity (antibodies that cause thyroid disease) who have manifestations of both hyperthyroidism and hypothyroidism. These can be patients who have both Graves' disease (autoimmune hyperthyroidism) and Hashimoto's thyroiditis (autoimmune hypothyroidism) simultaneously, meaning - at the same time. Some Hashimoto's patients experience this scenario short-term, which is called "Hashitoxicosis" but once the hyperthyroid phase subsides they will progress into hypothyroidism.

Some patients however continue this phasing back and forth which makes it difficult for most treating doctors who can neither treat the hyperthyroid or hypothyroid phases for fear that it will worsen one or the other. In some European countries, a treatment called "block and replace" is used to treat these type cases, which is a combination of using anti-thyroid drugs, followed by thyroid hormone replacement. It is a somewhat risky treatment that is not commonly used in the U.S. and therefore most doctors will instead refer the patient for a thyroidectomy or radioactive iodine destruction of the thyroid gland (ablation). Afterward, thyroid hormone replacement would be the treatment that follows.

Graves' Disease

This autoimmune cause of hyperthyroidism is often first treated using anti-thyroid drugs that slow production of thyroid hormones and/or beta-blocker drugs to control hyperthyroid symptoms. In many cases however, the drugs will need to be re-administered due to a return of the symptoms a few weeks or months following completion of the initial treatment phase. If after attempting to control the hyperthyroidism through reasonable trials of anti-thyroid medications, a patient will be referred for thyroidectomy or radioactive iodine ablation (RAI) if the initial treatments do not prove successful.

Another reason for first attempting to control the disease through drug therapies is the fact that RAI can increase the risk for development of Thyroid Eye Disease in some patients, especially in females, according to some medical information sources. If thyroid removal or ablation is performed, the patient will afterward need thyroid hormone replacement as a life long treatment. If the parathyroid glands are damaged during the procedure, calcium supplementation may also be necessary.

CHAPTER TWENTEIGHT

Temporary and Permanent Types of Thyroiditis

Inflammatory Thyroid Gland Conditions

Thyroiditis is a term meaning there is inflammation within the thyroid gland. There are types of this condition that are short-term and others that are life long.

When thyroiditis is permanent, this means a chronic disease process is being experienced directly within the gland. Temporary types of thyroiditis are those that are caused by pregnancy, illnesses or diseases indirectly affecting the thyroid gland (secondary causes).

Hashimoto's Thyroiditis

Hashimoto's, the most common type of chronic thyroiditis was discovered by a Japanese medical researcher, of the same name in 1912. It is an autoimmune condition that causes eventual progressive hypothyroidism (under-active thyroid) although in early stages of the disease, one can experience "Hashitoxicosis", intermittent and temporary phases of hyperthyroidism (overactive). The disease is characterized by antibodies that cause thyroid cell destruction that are detectable by blood lab testing. Some cases however are elusive to positive antibody readings and require an FNA (Fine Needle Tissue Biopsy) and/or a thyroid ultrasound for a definitive diagnosis.

Mild enlargement of the thyroid gland (goiter) is also common in Hashimoto's patients although in some patients goiters can be moderate to larger in size. Thyroid nodules, which are small tumorous growths in the gland, are also common with Hashimoto's.

Other Types of Permanent Thyroiditis

Other variants of permanent thyroiditis that are less common, include "Ord's thyroiditis", discovered 1877 in by Dr. Ord, which presents with the same auto-antibodies as Hashimoto's but results in progressive atrophy (shrinking) of the thyroid gland rather than goiter. Ord's is more common in European countries, while Hashimoto's is more common in the USA. Also "Riedel thyroiditis" (Riedel's Struma), discovered in 1883 by Dr. Riedel is a condition in which thyroid gland tissue is slowly replaced with fibrotic tissue (fibrosclerosis) and can extend beyond the thyroid gland into areas of the throat, posing danger of obstructed breathing and/or swallowing. Of the permanent types of thyroiditis, Riedels is the least common.

Temporary Sub-acute Thyroiditis

Sub-acute thyroiditis, also referred to as "de Quervain's thyroiditis" is a condition in which viral infections, usually of the respiratory type, are believed to settle into the thyroid gland, causing sudden high levels of inflammation (medical research continues in attempt to confirm the cause). The thyroid gland becomes painful in the case of sub-acute thyroiditis and patients who experience it will commonly run low-grade to moderate fevers. Once the immune system has fully eradicated the virus or other cause of the condition from the body, the thyroiditis will resolve within a few weeks following. Early into the onset of de Quervain's, patients may experience a phase of hyperthyroid symptoms.

Another Type of Temporary Thyroiditis

Following pregnancy, some women develop "Postpartum thyroiditis" which can occur as much as one year following giving birth. It is an inflammatory response within the thyroid gland and this type also manifests first with hyperthyroid symptoms. The condition will resolve in most patients, within three months although if it occurs in someone at high risk for thyroid autoimmunity (runs in their family), the condition can transition over to Hashimoto's and require lifelong treatment of hypothyroidism. Since the condition can occur apart from pregnancies and in male patients, it is also referred to as "Silent thyroiditis", meaning it does not cause pain in the thyroid gland as Sub-acute thyroiditis does.

Treatments

If thyroiditis is permanent and causes thyroid hormone imbalance, this will require thyroid hormone replacement therapy if hypothyroidism develops or anti-thyroid drugs and/or beta-blockers, if hyperthyroidism develops. Some diseased thyroid glands may need to be partially or fully removed by surgical thyroidectomy or destroyed by radioactive iodine ablation. In the case of temporary thyroiditis, most patients will require no treatment but will simply be prescribed bed-rest until the condition resolves over a few weeks.

For those who develop severe inflammation, corticosteroids (steroid anti-inflammatory drugs) may be prescribed for short term use. If fever is present, over-the-counter fever-reducing drugs may need to be taken, such as aspirin or ibuprofen.

CHAPTER TWENTYNINE

The T3 and T4 Thyroid Hormone Blood Tests

Understanding Your Lab Results

Thyroid blood testing is used to diagnose thyroid hormone disorders and diseases. They are also used to monitor thyroid hormone treatments.

The major thyroid hormones, T4 and T3 can be directly measured in the blood as can the pituitary hormone called TSH (Thyroid Stimulating Hormone) that reflects the levels of thyroid hormones. Blood testing is highly accurate and is the most common form of testing to diagnose thyroid disorders.

Thyroxine-T4

This metabolism-regulating hormone manufactured by the thyroid gland is the most abundant in the body but is less powerful than the T3 hormone (to be addressed in a later subheading). The ratio of T4 compared to T3 is approximately 75% T4 to 25% T3. Thyroxine-T4 is a reserve hormone that remains on standby (precursor) to be converted into Triiodothyronine-T3, the hormone most responsible for metabolism-regulation as needed in the body. Any surplus of the T4 that is not used-up during the conversion process is instead converted into a substance called Reverse-T3, which means it has been rendered inactive, so that any excess does not remain in the body and cause an overactive metabolism or "hyperthyroidism".

T4 Blood Tests

Blood tests that measure the T4 come in a variety of versions, including the "Total T4" (also called Thyroxine), the "Free T4" (considered the best by some specialists) and the "Free Thyroxine Index" (FTI). All of the tests that help determine the T4 level in the body have lab ranges (normal values) with a flagged-high reading indicating hyperthyroidism and a flagged-low reading indicating hypothyroidism.

If for example the T4 has a reference range at a testing lab of "4.0 to 12.0", a reading above 12.0 is suggestive of an overactive thyroid gland. A reading below 4.0 would be suggestive of an under-active thyroid gland. High-normal or low-normal readings and those that are borderline, are also suspect for developing thyroid hormone disorders and merit follow up retesting. Thyroid doctors who treat thyroid hormone imbalances use a narrowed therapy treatment goal that would keep the T4 level at approximately between mid range and higher normal.

Triiodothyronine-T3

This thyroid hormone comes directly from the T4 via the conversion process previously mentioned, unless administered orally from an outside source. The T4 accomplishes this by dropping one iodine atom from its molecules which transforms it into the more metabolically active T3. Medical sources state that the manufactured T3 is about five times more powerful than T4 in regulating the metabolism.

In certain types of hypothyroidism, the T3 will go low while the T4 level remains normal. There are a variety of names for this type hypothyroidism but all can be referred to under the term "Low T3 Syndrome". The condition is often diagnosed by measuring the blood-level of Reverse T3 in the body, which becomes highly elevated when there is a normal amount of T4 that is not being converted into enough T3 to support metabolism.

T3 Blood Tests

This hormone is also ordered in either the "Total" or "Free" level and just like the T4, a result that is elevated above normal, points to a diagnosis of hyperthyroidism, while a below normal result points to hypothyroidism. T3 is usually tested in combination with T4 and TSH and is rarely tested alone unless a patient with Low T3 Syndrome is being treated with T3-only replacement hormone therapy.

The normal range for Total T3 is approximately "80 to 225" and the normal range for Free T3 is approximately "2.0 to 4.0". Above normal readings help to diagnose cases of hyperthyroidism and below normal readings help to diagnoses hypothyroidism.

T3 Resin Uptake Test

One blood test that is sometimes included on thyroid panels is the "T3 Resin Uptake". This test should not be confused with those that measure T3 levels in the body. This test instead, measures how well the blood uptakes the T3 hormone. A patient's blood sample has T3 added to it at the lab and if uptake of the hormone into the blood for use in the cells and tissues of the body, is hindered (not adequate), this helps to determine a disease process that is blocking this action.

Autoimmune thyroid diseases that present with auto-antibodies that attack thyroid proteins can be a cause of a low T3 Resin Uptake. One type of thyroid antibody that can hinder T3 from up-taking in the blood, is the one that attacks "thyroxine-binding globulin" (TBG) called "anti-TBG antibodies". TBG is the protein that binds with thyroxine in the blood stream, so that it can enter receptor-cells and tissues and convert into T3 as needed. High or low levels of T3 Uptake can mean different things depending upon how it compares with thyroid hormone levels and the level of TBG itself.

CHAPTER THIRTY

Is Iodine a Safe Thyroid Supplement?

Keeping Iodine in its Proper Place

Iodine is an essential element needed for proper thyroid function. In some thyroid disease cases however, iodine supplementation may be contraindicated (risks involved).

Many companies that manufacture supplements advertised to boost thyroid function often place high levels of iodine content in them or include ingredients that are rich in iodine, such as kelp (seaweed-algae). While reasonable levels of iodine intake is healthy for people with non-diseased thyroid glands, it can have adverse effects in some cases when thyroid disease is present or if other thyroid treatments are already being administered.

Iodine for Treating Hypothyroidism

The only hypothyroid condition, in which iodine is administered as the treatment, is iodine deficiency hypothyroidism. The condition is not common in industrialized countries that have iodized table salt and healthy iodine-rich foods available. Endemic goiters caused by low iodine are a feature of the condition and medical lab testing can also help to identify it.

If hypothyroidism is from any other cause, thyroid hormone replacement will be the prescribed treatment. A diseased thyroid gland or one not properly regulated by the endocrine brain-glands (central hypothyroidism) cannot be restored to normal function through iodine replacement therapy. Thyroid hormone is what is missing in these cases and there is no substitute for replacement hormone therapy.

Iodine Adverse in Combination with Thyroid Hormone Therapy

When thyroid hormone is taken orally, this replaces the thyroid gland's job in manufacturing thyroid hormone from iodine. It can no longer perform this function due to a disease process in the gland or dysfunction of other endocrine glands that regulate the thyroid as mentioned previously. Taking iodine supplements in addition to a thyroid hormone dose could have adverse effects because a diseased thyroid is unable to absorb the surplus of iodine.

As a result, the levels of added iodine may become abnormally high in the blood stream, causing a toxic reaction in the body. In addition to this, it may also affect the stability of a thyroid hormone dose and cause monitored levels of the hypothyroid therapy to be less accurate on blood retests.

Iodine Toxicity

Excessive iodine intake is a direct cause of thyroid disease according to some researchers. In medical studies regarding iodine supplementation, it has been found that abnormally high levels can increase the risk for developing conditions of thyroid autoimmunity (autoimmune thyroiditis). These would be the diseases that cause the immune system to attack the thyroid gland via auto-antibodies that destroy the proteins in the gland responsible for converting iodine into thyroid hormone. It may be that the body detects the risk for thyrotoxicity (hyperthyroidism) from highly elevated iodine levels and as a result, turns against the thyroid gland in attempt to halt the onset of thyroid hormone imbalance.

Additionally, patients scheduled for radioactive iodine uptake scans or who are hyperthyroid and scheduled for radioactive iodine ablation of their thyroid glands (removal by tissue destruction) are asked to remove all iodine from their diets. This no-iodine or in some cases low-iodine (reduced but not eliminated) diet recommendation prescribed by treating doctors depends on each individual thyroid disease case.

These facts point to the importance in thyroid patients discussing with their doctors what role iodine plays in their particular case and in also informing their doctors about any supplement they may be taking that contains iodine, even if it is only trace amounts found in a multi-vitamin.

CHAPTER THIRTYONE

Conditions Related to Hashimoto's Thyroiditis

Complications from Thyroid Autoimmunity

Hashitoxicosis and Hashimoto's Encephalopathy are potentially serious conditions associated with Hashimoto's thyroiditis that require specific treatments.

Hashimoto's thyroiditis, an autoimmune disease of the thyroid gland that causes eventual hypothyroidism, can potentially cause other related conditions. Some of these possible complications are more common than others and some can be severe or even life threatening but each of them have treatments available once they are recognized and diagnosed. In the subheadings below, the related conditions called "Hashitoxicosis" and "Hashimoto's Encephalopathy" will be addressed.

Hashitoxicosis

Some patients with Hashimoto's thyroiditis, experience phases of hyperthyroidism, before progressive hypothyroidism sets in. These spells of hyperthyroid symptoms are referred to as Hashitoxicosis and the condition can cause moderate to full-blown hyperthyroidism that is short term. If these phases were not short term but permanent and progressive, a diagnosis of Graves' disease (autoimmune caused hyperthyroidism) would instead be given.

The cause of Hashitoxicosis is the same as in other hyperthyroid conditions and that is an abnormally high increase in thyroid hormone levels. While some medical sources state that this condition is not common, it may be more common in less severe cases and mild manifestations of Hashitoxicosis may be responsible for anxiety symptoms in some patients.

The cause and Manifestation of Hashitoxicosis

There are two medical opinions as to why these hyperthyroid phases occur before hypothyroidism takes over. One being, that it occurs in some Hashimoto's patients who are mildly positive for "TSI" antibodies (Thyroid Stimulating Immunoglobulins) that typically cause Graves' disease hyperthyroidism.

The second being that thyroid gland cell-death from the antibodies found in higher titers in Hashimoto's patients (anti-TPO and Anti-TG) cause release of stored hormone from these dying cells at a faster rate, early into the onset of hypothyroidism. Once this faster phase of cell death levels-off to a slower rate, due to the thyroid gland being unable to generate new cells as quickly, hypothyroidism will then take over.

During the hyperthyroid phases, a patient will experience hyperthyroid symptoms including, nervousness, trembling, sweating, increased bowel movements and temporary rapid weight loss.

Treatment for Hashitoxicosis

If a Hashimoto's patient is already taking thyroid hormone replacement, a treating doctor may need to discontinue their thyroid dose if Hashitoxicosis is experienced. The patient would also need monitored to make sure the hyperthyroid phase is not a permanent transition over to Graves' disease. Short-term use of a low-dose beta-blocker or anti-thyroid medication might also be administered and/or an anti-anxiety medication.

Rarely some patients do continue to phase back and forth between hypothyroidism and hyperthyroidism and in these cases it becomes difficult to administer either thyroid hormone replacement or anti-thyroid drugs. Highly skilled thyroid specialists may chose to administer a combination of both, which is referred to as "block and replace" however, in most cases of highly unstable thyroid function, the patient is referred for thyroidectomy (surgical thyroid removal) or radioactive iodine destruction of the gland (ablation).

Hashimoto's Encephalopathy

The majority of Hashimoto's patients test positive for thyroid antibodies, the killer cells created by the immune system to attack thyroid proteins that are responsible for the manufacture of thyroid hormone from iodine. While this is a misdirected immune response that causes damage to thyroid gland cells, it occurs due to an incorrect recognition of these natural thyroid cells as threats within the body.

As this auto-antibody attack occurs, the body produces an inflammatory response that can contribute to a goiter and according to some medical research opinions, can also contribute to rheumatic symptoms in the body, affecting joints and muscles.

With Hashimoto's Encephalopathy, this inflammatory response to these antibodies called the anti-thyroidperoxidase/Anti-TPO, also referred to as "anti-microsomal antibodies", causes severe inflammation that begins affecting the brain. While the condition is very rare, it can occur in Hashimoto's patients who are only sub-clinically hypothyroid or even those who are euthyroid (normal hormone levels).

Symptoms of Hashimoto's Encephalopathy

For reasons not fully understood, these high levels of inflammation, affect tissues and nerves in the brain that control motor responses and other brain-signals sent throughout the body. The resulting symptoms of interrupted brain function can result in severe neurological symptoms, including difficulty with walking and speech, involuntary movements, seizures, psychotic episodes (hallucinations and delusions) and stroke type symptoms. Without treatment, brain damage will occur and eventual coma or death may result as well. It is an emergency situation and treatment must be administered immediately once Hashimoto's Encephalopathy has been recognized and diagnosed.

Treatment for Hashimoto's Encephalopathy

Treatment for this inflammatory condition is by administering corticosteroid drugs to reduce the inflammation affecting the brain. These drugs are a type of synthetic cortisol steroid that is commonly available in the brand name Prednisone. The drug is usually only required for a two to three week period and will bring down the inflammation and resolve the neurological symptoms. Some patients require no further treatment once the initial drug therapy is completed while others may need the corticosteroid treatment repeated if the condition relapses.

CHAPTER THIRTYTWO

Mild Adrenal Insufficiency in Thyroid Disease

Why Thyroid Patients Experience Adrenal Fatigue

Adrenal Fatigue is experienced in thyroid patients before treatment but the inflammatory effect of thyroid autoimmunity may also contribute to an ongoing adrenal problem.

Mild adrenal insufficiency or "Adrenal Fatigue" has been found in medical research studies, to occur in a number of chronic diseases and inflammatory conditions. These include asthma, Post Traumatic Stress Disorder, inflammatory bowel diseases and rheumatic diseases affecting the muscles and/or joints (i.e., fibromyalgia and rheumatoid arthritis).

The mild adrenal insufficient states found in these conditions, were concluded by the findings of low DHEA (dehydroepiandrosterone) and/or low cortisol (adrenocortical), the two major adrenal hormones that regulate sex hormone production, stress coping and anti-inflammatory responses in the body.

Adrenal Fatigue and Thyroid Disease

While thyroid disease is not often mentioned in medical studies, as a condition that can result in mild adrenal insufficiency, low adrenal function is listed as a potential symptom of hypothyroidism on many medical information sources. If the hypothyroidism has "thyroid autoimmunity" as the cause this places further demand on the under-functioning adrenal glands which serve as part of their purpose, the moderating of inflammation in the body, via the natural anti-inflammatory properties of the hormone-cortisol.

Hypothyroidism and Slowed Adrenal Function

When a patient experiences the onset of hypothyroidism, all organs in the body also begin to hypo-function, including the endocrine glands. The adrenals also being a part of the endocrine system can be affected resulting is slowed hormone output from them as well. The endocrine system as a whole, works in synchronization and the thyroid glands depend on the adrenal cortisol hormone, which aids in converting T4 thyroid hormone into the more metabolically active T3.

Some medical researchers also believe that cortisol helps thyroid hormone to perform its metabolic-regulating effect on the tissues and cells of the body. Medical sources who do recognize and study mild adrenal insufficiency, state that Adrenal Fatigue occurs after a hyper-functioning phase of the adrenal glands. Any condition including chronic stress, disease or inflammatory response in the body, places an abnormally high demand on the adrenal glands for cortisol output, which can be followed by a fatigue-stage or what might be referred to as "exhausted adrenal reserves".

Autoimmune Thyroid Disease and Inflammation

The majority of thyroid disease patients in industrialized countries, experience the resulting hypothyroid or hyperthyroid conditions, due to "thyroid autoimmunity". As mentioned previously, thyroid diseases of this type cause an inflammatory response in the thyroid gland. This requires a response from the adrenal glands, to send more cortisol to moderate the inflammation that occurs due to the autoimmune response. The immune system is creating auto-antibodies, sent to attack thyroid proteins that are mistakenly recognized as invaders in the body that need to be destroyed.

As thyroid tissue begins to become damaged and as its cells begin to die, inflammation develops in the gland. This can occur even before thyroid hormone levels become imbalanced, evident by the fact that autoimmune thyroid patients often develop goiters (thyroid swelling) in advance of hypothyroid or hyperthyroid hormone levels.

These facts demonstrate that thyroid disease can create a high demand for cortisol output by the adrenals. It would seem obvious that this would result in mild adrenal insufficient states in some thyroid patients, especially those whose adrenal function is less sufficient than that of the average healthy person.

CHAPTER THIRTYTHREE

Being a Proactive Thyroid Patient

Sharing Knowledge and Personal Experience

Thyroid patients can benefit a great deal from the experiences and basic knowledge shared by other patients and being proactive can be done in-balance.

Being a pro-active thyroid patient simply means one is actively involved in following the best plan for better health that comes from knowledge received through search and treatment experiences. It also means a patient is being fully cooperative with his doctor and offering the input needed that can help him receive best possible treatment.

Partnering with Your Doctor

Recently the U.S. National Institutes of Health has been airing a radio commercial, recommending that patients with treated health conditions become more proactive in their own medical care. Their advice includes becoming a partner with the doctors by being as communicative with them as possible, being fully descriptive about any changes in symptoms or concerns that might arise in regard to treatment. They include the suggestion in the ad that patients take notes and carry the notes with them to their doctor office visits.

Unfortunately, some opinions you find online and elsewhere contradicts this opinion and rather suggests that patients place all responsibility for their health care upon their doctors and that they should offer no input as a treated patient. Common sense says however that it can only be a benefit to both the patient and doctor if a patient offers a reasonable amount of input in regard to his case and this can only be done if there is a degree of education on the part of the patient in regard to his illness and the treatment being administered for it.

Helping Educate Other Thyroid Patients

Each January is "Thyroid Awareness Month" and patients are encouraged to help get the word out about thyroid diseases, their symptoms and the tests that can diagnose them. The American Thyroid Association (ATA) for example, that offers resources for both patients and doctors, offers educational brochures for patients that can be printed and shared or that patients can share the online links to. This campaign has a number of medical societies involved including the ATA and the American College of Endocrinologists (ACE) and has as its goal, the better educating of the general public about thyroid diseases and disorders.

The reason these medical societies see the necessity of this campaign, is due to the fact that they have estimated that up to half of people with thyroid disease remain undiagnosed. The two reasons this occurs is due to a lack of public education and a lack of detailed communication by patients to their doctors. In addition to Thyroid Awareness Month, the ACE has also published an online magazine available free to the public called "Power of Prevention" (POP), in which they help the public become better educated about endocrine diseases, with some of the segments being designed for educating children.

Sharing Your Story and Basic Knowledge

Thyroid patients benefit from hearing a fellow-patient's story because it is someone they can relate-to, having gone through similar experiences to theirs. Some thyroid disease cases can present with severe symptoms and some require surgeries to correct and these aspects can make patients feel somewhat isolated in their experience from their healthy family, friends and co-workers. A feeling of support can come from reading other patients' stories that include their symptom struggles, difficulties adjusting to treatments and their treatment successes. This is especially true in patients who have cases of thyroid cancer.

Sharing basic knowledge a thyroid patient has learned can be done on thyroid disease patient-forums, in online articles and in printed books. This presents the question as to what a patient can reasonably write about when sharing their knowledge in articles or forum posts. The answer to this question would be that any information that can be well-confirmed should be acceptable between thyroid patients sharing knowledge and that they may offer to the general public.

Obviously if information is basic and found on many sources easily confirmed by search, these type articles should not require confirmation of the facts. If however a point is made in an article that involves areas of controversy or that includes more advanced medical knowledge, confirming sources should be cited that are reputable and reliable.

If even the basic points in a thyroid patient article require confirmation, this can add unnecessary length to it and actually serve to confuse the reader. It should therefore be determined as to which information is basic enough to be easily confirmed and that which is more complicated and in need of citing confirming sources.

CHAPTER THIRTYFOUR

Online Thyroid Support and Information

Coping For Patients on the World Wide Web

Thyroid patients can be profoundly affected by symptoms and changes to their lives that thyroid disease can bring but there are helpful online coping-resources available.

The internet contains a wonderful source of helpful information and places of support offered to patients suffering chronic diseases, including thyroid-related ones. Patients suffering under-active and overactive thyroid disorder symptoms can connect to fellow patients and become self-educated about the disease that is affecting their lives.

Thyroid Patient Advocate Information Sites

There are a large number of dependable and reputable information sources online that supply helpful information that can be relied upon. There are a number of well-informed writers that offer information on a full range of thyroid related subjects. You'll find articles on reputable websites on hyperthyroid, hypothyroid, and thyroid autoimmunity conditions and about symptom manifestations that are experienced with these disorders.

Many of the writers of online thyroid disease information are also fellow thyroid patients or what are also referred to as "Thyroid Patient Advocates". There are website information sources by well-studied patient advocates who are also well recognized authors of best selling books on thyroid subjects, including Elaine Moore and Mary Shomon. Patients can take advantage of the great information offered by these and other authors, both online and by obtaining their books in print.

Medical Thyroid Information Sites

These type sites offer information from a purely medical standpoint, without the fellow-patient view but can also be greatly instrumental in helping thyroid patients become better educated about their disorders. While doctors can help patients gain a general understanding about their conditions, they seldom have the time needed to fully educate their patients as they desire to be. Learning about a disease that is often life-long and that can cause a degree of change in activity and lifestyle by patients who suffer them, can help take away some of the fear and uncertainty from the experience, especially in newly diagnosed patients.

Medical thyroid information sites that can be helpful to patients include the American Thyroid Association, Thyroid Disease Manager and the American Thyroid Association (patient brochures).

Patient Blogs and Forums

Many patients have blogs online, where they post ongoing information about their personal experience with thyroid disease. Other patients reading their posts can find experiences they relate to, that can help them feel less alone with their disease. Some blogs also allow posting via message boards or forums that are available on their pages. Other forums and message boards are for the sole purpose of posting thyroid-related questions and for fellow-patient information sharing and support. Some are also moderated by volunteer medical professionals who reply to patient's questions.

An online search using Google or other search engines, including the keywords "thyroid blogs", "personal thyroid stories" and "thyroid forums and message boards", will yield many pages showing the available resources in these areas. Thyroid patients who feel the need for support and/or information can take advantage of these type resources and if they do not own a computer, can go online free of charge at a public library.

(END)

www.ingramcontent.com/pod-product-compliance
Lightning Source LLC
Chambersburg PA
CBHW020412290526
45785CB00002B/520